BRADY
EKG Technician

Roberta C. Weiss, LVN, Ed.D.
Allied Health Curriculum Specialist
Teacher Trainer, UCLA Education Extension Division

8/07

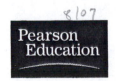

BRADY
PRENTICE HALL CAREER & TECHNOLOGY
PRENTICE HALL, Upper Saddle River, New Jersey 07458

Library of Congress Cataloging-in-Publication Data

Weiss, Roberta C.
    The EKG technician / Roberta C. Weiss.
      p. cm.
    ISBN 0-89303-702-8
    1. Electrocardiography. 2. Medical technology. I. Title.
    [DNLM: 1. Allied Health Personnel—education.
2. Electrocardiography. WG 140 W432e]
RC683.5.E5 W38 1990
616.1′207547—dc20
DNLM/DLC
for Library of Congress   89-70794
                                                        CIP

Editorial/production supervision and
   interior design: Ed Jones
Cover design: Santora
Manufacturing buyer: Dave Dickey
Photo credit: FPG International;
   photographer: T. Tracy

©1990 by Prentice-Hall, Inc.
   A Pearson Education Company
   Upper Saddle River, NJ 07458

Printed in the United States of America

15 14

ISBN 0-89303-702-8

Prentice-Hall International (UK) Limited,London
Prentice-Hall of Australia Pty. Limited, Sydney
Prentice-Hall Canada Inc., Toronto
Prentice-Hall Hispanoamericana, S.A., Mexico
Prentice-Hall of India Private Limited, New Delhi
Prentice-Hall of Japan, Inc., Tokyo
Pearson Education Asia Pte. Ltd., Singapore
Editora Prentice-Hall do Brasil, Ltda., Rio de Janeiro

DEDICATION

*This textbook is dedicated, with love and respect,
to Ms. Marla Keeth, LVN, a "teacher's teacher,"
for all of her love, abundant support, patience, understanding,
and great desire to help teach all of the students
who are fortunate enough to come her way.*

Contents

Preface

This book is written in simple language, and is accompanied by basic illustrations, in order to provide the reader with a well-rounded introduction to the principles and techniques involved in working as an EKG technician.

While the author believes there are many adequate textbooks currently in use that provide the learner with advanced techniques and interpretation of electrocardiograms, it is the goal of this manual to present the student with the "basics" necessary to function as a valued member of the health care delivery team.

The text is divided into 14 chapters, beginning with basic concepts of electrocardiography and concluding with surgical and advanced interventions for the cardiac patient. In addition, the text also addresses understanding and recording of vital signs as well as performing cardiopulmonary resuscitation.

To assist readers in understanding the subject matter, each chapter is accompanied by terminal and competency objectives at the beginning and review questions at the end.

Two appendices provide practice sheets and answers for the interpretation of EKG tracings. A third appendix gives the answers to the end-of-chapter review questions. A series of tear-out flashcards, following the index, is also provided, to help the student interpret different arrhythmias.

Roberta C. Weiss, LVN, Ed.D.
Van Nuys, California

Acknowledgments

I want to extend my deepest gratitude and appreciation to all those who have assisted me in the preparation and development of this textbook, including:

Ms. Phyllis Stilson, RN, my past nursing instructor and dearest friend, who provided me with the "basics" necessary in the delivery of health care for all patients

All of my teachers and professors in health care, education, and journalism who provided me with the skills and concepts necessary to write this book

Robyn Gilmore, a talented artist, and friend for almost 40 years, who worked around the clock for three days and nights, helping to formulate sketches for illustrations for this text

All EKG technician students, past and present, who showed me there was a need to develop a text simple enough to meet their individual needs

Ms. Gretchen Spence, National Director of Education for Concord Career colleges, for all of her feedback in delineating the needs of the EKG technician student

Mr. Mike Robison, equipment specialist for Mission Medical Supply, Inc., for all his help in providing me information regarding the different types of EKG machines currently in use

Finally, I want to thank Mr. Matt McNearney, Health Occupations Editor, for all of his help, understanding, cooperation, and, particularly, his willingness to take a chance on me.

Introduction to Electrocardiography

1

TERMINAL OBJECTIVE

To introduce the student to the study of electrocardiography through a brief history of the concept and identification of the members of the electrocardiography department.

COMPETENCY OBJECTIVES

Upon completion of this chapter, the student will be able to:

1. Correctly spell and define terminology related to the study of electrocardiography.
2. Give a brief account of the history of electrocardiography.
3. Describe the various careers and personnel who may work in the EKG department.
4. Describe the duties and responsibilities of the EKG technician.
5. Briefly explain the educational requirements of the EKG technician.
6. List some of the personal characteristics and qualities desirable for the EKG technician.

HISTORY OF ELECTROCARDIOGRAPHY

Before we can go on to learn about the role or function of the electro-cardiograph technician, it is important that you grasp how this precise measurement of the heart's function first came about.

The association of electricity with the heart's muscle activity, or what is more commonly known as *electrocardiography,* has been known for more than 200 years; however, it was not until the end of the nineteenth century that quantitative measurement of muscle electricity even became a possibility. Earlier, there was no instrument (or what is now referred to as a *galvanometer)* sensitive enough to detect the extremely small electrical signals associated with muscle contraction. In the case of the human heart, the problem was magnified by the fact that measurements had to be made on the surface of the body, where the signal was greatly attenuated.

Though several earlier devices were developed, the first practical recording galvanometer sensitive enough to detect the electrocardiograph was developed in Holland in 1903 by an electrical scientist by the name of William Einthoven. Einthoven's instrument, termed a "string galvanometer," consisted of an extremely fine quartz wire, much finer than a human hair, which was suspended between the poles of a powerful electromagnet. The wire was made conductive, or electrically active, by coating it with a fine layer of silver, whose ends were connected to the patient. The minute currents that would flow through the wire, resulting from the heart's electrical voltages, then caused it to deflect slightly into the magnetic field. Finally, a beam of light, which was focused onto the wire, would then cast a shadow that was magnified and projected onto a photographic plate.

Over a period of time, Einthoven communicated his discovery to his friend, Sir Horace Darwin, founder of the Cambridge Scientific Instrument Company, located in England, as well as to Professor Horalto Williams, in the United States. However, when representatives of both scientists visited Einthoven, they soon discovered that his original instrument was so bulky that it occupied two rooms and needed five people to operate it. Although both scientests indicated that the size of Einthoven's "electrical instrument" was much too large to warrant their involvement in its manufacture, based on scientific papers published by Einthoven, they did believe it demonstrated some dramatic medical benefits. Therefore, although Darwin's feelings about development of the instrument still remained "lukewarm," he also believed its manufacture could eventually assist the medical community in measuring the heart's electrical impulses. Based on this notion, he contracted with

Einthoven to transform his invention into a more practical, commercial instrument.

Meanwhile, in the United States, Professor Williams and his assistant, Charles Hindle, had already begun work on their own instrument. By 1922, the two scientists merged with Darwin's Cambridge Company and have since continued their joint development and manufacturing of what came to be known as electrocardiograph machines.

Though considered a major improvement over Einthoven's original model, the first Cambridge electrocardiograph machine weighed over 350 pounds. By 1930, after modifications were made to reduce its size, a compact instrument, weighing 30 pounds, was eventually produced. The original carbon arc lamp was replaced by a filament bulb, and the glass photographic plate was changed to a sheet film. The galvanometer itself eventually became greatly reduced in size, including the clumsy porcelain pot electrodes that were replaced by small plates of nickel-silver alloy.

While major changes had occurred in the actual size of the instrument, the next major advance was to employ a thermionic vacuum tube amplifier that would amplify the electrocardiograph signal, thereby making it so powerful that it would drive a direct-writing galvanometer.

Once the size of the instrument had been greatly reduced, discovery of the transistor's use in its manufacture was only a few years away. By the late 1940s, the use of what has come to be known as the solid-state electronic electrocardiographic instrument began to be commercially produced, evolving into what many physicians have come to depend upon for the measurement of the electrical impulses on the human heart. (See Figure 1–1.)

DEFINING THE ELECTROCARDIOGRAPH TRACING

Before we can even begin to understand the purpose of the electrocardiograph and the role the electrocardiograph technician plays in securing this scientific measurement, it is extremely important that you understand what exactly an electrocardiographic tracing represents.

An electrocardiographic tracing, sometimes referred to as an EKG or ECG, utilizes an electronic device, called an electrocardiographic machine, in order to measure or record the electrical charges that occur during a complete heartbeat. These recordings help the physician to diagnose any irregularities or changes in the patient's heart action, and they are usually performed routinely as the patient ages as well as before or after surgery, and as a diagnostic tool in assisting the physician in caring for the patient. (See Figures 1–2 and 1–3.)

THE EKG DEPARTMENT

While many physicians perform electrocardiograms in their office, the majority are done in the hospital or in outpatient facilities or clinics. In the hospital, the EKG department may be housed as a separate unit or as part of another department. Many smaller hospitals, for example, house

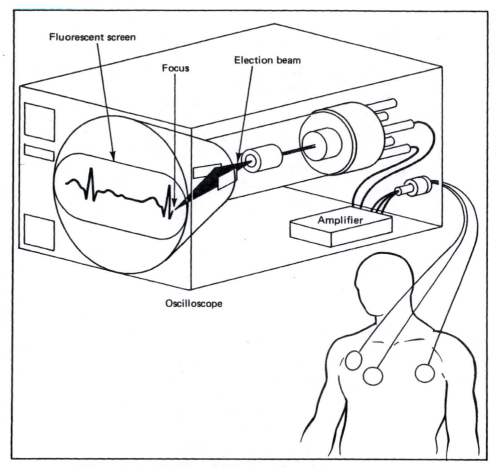

Figure 1—1 The use of the oscilloscope as a means of recording the electrocardiogram.

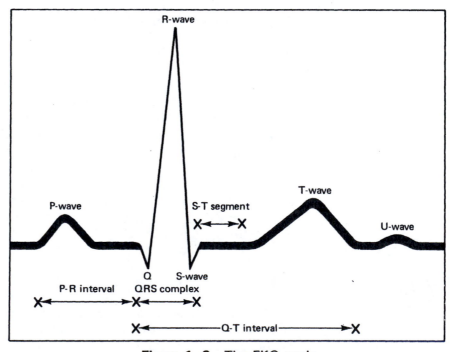

Figure 1—2 The EKG cycle.

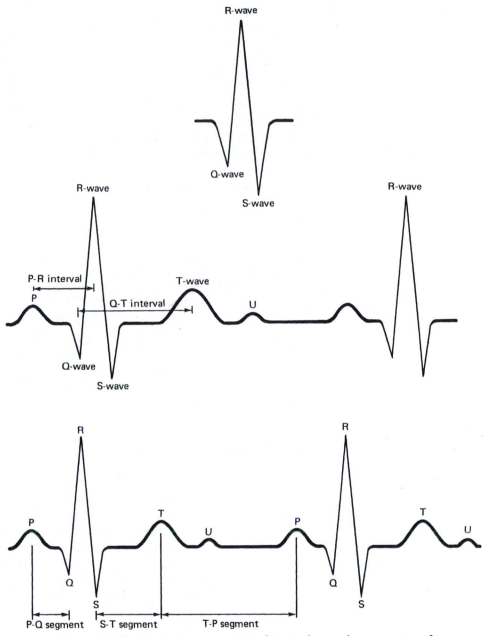

Figure 1–3 Complexes, waves, intervals, and segments of the electrocardiogram.

both their respiratory therapy and their EKG units in one combined area, often referred to as the *cardiopulmonary department*.

MEMBERS OF THE EKG DEPARTMENT

Both the size of the department and the number of EKGs performed will greatly affect the number of people associated with the EKG department. In most large medical facilities, such as hospitals and medical centers, there are usually four levels of career ladder positions found within the EKG department. These levels include the EKG Technician I, the EKG Technician II, the Cardiovascular Technician, and the Cardiologist, or the medical doctor responsible for overseeing the entire department. In addition to these four major positions, there may also be other members of the staff whose role is related or more specialized but who may also be considered members of the EKG department. These include a Treadmill Technician, a Holter Recorder Scanning Technician, an Echocardiograph Technician, and a Cardiac Catheterization Technician.

The Cardiovascular Technician

The role of the cardiovascular technician involves the responsibility of analyzing arterial and venous blood bases and acid-based variables. This individual is also responsible for collecting respiratory gases and operating certain equipment, as well as performing certain invasive and noninvasive procedures, including any emergency therapeutic procedures, as the situation may warrant.

In addition to working within the EKG department, the cardiovascular technician may also be a member of the cardiac catheterization laboratory, the coronary care or intensive care unit, and the emergency room department. When not required to perform certain diagnostic and invasive and noninvasive tests, this person's primary responsibility is to be on standby as a member of the coronary or heart emergency care team, and to assist during any emergency situations that might arise.

The Cardiologist

As we have already stated, a cardiologist is a medical doctor specializing in the care and treatment of patients with conditions affecting the heart and the cardiovascular system. This individual is responsible for both ordering and interpreting all medical tests that might be necessary for the accurate diagnosis and treatment of heart disorders. The cardiologist is also responsible for overseeing the smooth performance of the EKG equipment, and in many case the coronary care, intensive care, and emergency room departments of a large hospital.

The EKG Technician

The EKG technician, working under the direction of a cardiology supervisor or cardiologist, is responsible for performing routine EKGs as well as any procedures related to the position (as defined by the facility in which the technician works) as well as the training which the technician has completed. This individual is also responsible for operating certain equipment utilized in the performance of the position as well as performing certain tests that may be necessary for patient treatment within the hospital or in the medical office or clinic.

Responsibilities of the EKG technician may vary according to the level of training and the environment in which he or she is employed;

however, there are certain tasks that all EKG technicians are expected to perform. These include preparing patients for testing, operating the electrocardiograph machine, and recording the 12-lead EKG rhythm strips in a manner that provides reliable tests for the physician's interpretation. Other responsibilities include cutting and mounting the EKG strips; retrieving previous EKG recordings and attaching the new tracings to the patient's chart; filing paperwork as may be required; maintaining equipment and ordering supplies; preparing copies of a patient's EKG tracing; distributing original EKG reports for patient's charts and copies to physician's offices; forwarding charges for services to billing departments; and notifying a supervisor immediately of any deviations from a patient's normal or average EKG reading.

CHARACTERISTICS, TRAINING, AND EMPLOYMENT OF THE EKG TECHNICIAN

As in any other allied health position, training and securing an education as an EKG technician are only two aspects of becoming a valued member of the health care team. While the educational requirements usually include being either a high school graduate, or passing a GED equivalency test upon entrance into an EKG technician program, as well as successfully completing a vocational training program in this area, certain other characteristics and personality traits are necessary for the graduate to be successful in this position. These include the ability to communicate clearly in order to explain certain procedures to patients; the ability to coordinate both eye and hand movements in order to record the electrocardiogram; and proper finger dexterity, necessary to attach electrodes and operate equipment.

The EKG technician should also be someone who not only has a genuine desire to work with people but who is also interested in the technical and scientific information as it relates to understanding the significance of the EKG testing and its relationship to the patient's anatomy and physiology, particularly the heart's action.

The technician should also have the ability to work well under pressure, oftentimes in an emergency, as well as be able to deal with people and gain their cooperation. This person must have an even temperament, for much of the work required of the technician oftentimes requires day-after-day routine tasks.

Once the EKG technician has completed a prescribed course of study and exhibited signs of being a mature, caring person, there is no limit to the opportunities available to this individual in the health care field. Technicians are employed in both general and acute-care hospitals and medical centers; in skilled nursing facilities and extended-care facilities; in clinics, outpatient centers, and urgent-care facilities; and in private medical practices and physician's offices.

REVIEW QUESTIONS

Directions: For the questions below, give the answers you believe are most correct:

1. Who was responsible for developing the first practical recording galvanometer sensitive enough to detect the electrocardiograph?

2. What is the purpose of recording an electrocardiogram?

3. List three levels on the career ladder available to the EKG technician:

    (a) _____

    (b) _____

    (c) _____

4. List three related and specialized areas of the EKG Department:

    (a) _____

    (b) _____

    (c) _____

5. Put an "X" before each duty you will perform as an EKG technician:

    _____ Operate the EKG machine

    _____ Assist with a heart catheterization

    _____ Administer heart medications

    _____ Cut and mount EKG strips

    _____ Consult with the physician

    _____ Maintain EKG equipment

    _____ Forward charges for services to billing department

    _____ Prepare copies of EKG strips

    _____ Order supplies

    _____ Notify supervisor immediately of deviations from normal on an EKG recording

6. List at least five personal characteristics/traits an EKG technician should possess:

    (a) _____

    (b) _____

    (c) _____

    (d) _____

    (e) _____

7. List three areas in which an EKG technician may be employed:

    (a) _____

    (b) _____

    (c) _____

8. EKG technician training is generally completed through a _____

    _____ program.

Terminology and Electrocardiography

2

TERMINAL OBJECTIVE

To provide the student with an understanding of the terms, abbreviations, and symbols associated with the study of electrocardiography.

COMPETENCY OBJECTIVES

Upon completion of this chapter, the student will be able to

1. Identify and describe the fundamentals of medical terminology.
2. Discuss the importance of spelling and punctuation and the role each plays in medical terminology.
3. List the guidelines for proper identification and spelling of medical terms.
4. Discuss the concept of forming plural endings.
5. Correctly spell and define words, symbols, and abbreviations most frequently associated with the study of electrocardiography.

UNDERSTANDING THE PRINCIPLES OF MEDICAL TERMINOLOGY

Before we can begin to discuss some of the more frequently used terms and abbreviations acceptable in the study of electrocardiography, it is important that we spend a few moments reviewing some of the basic principles and concepts involved in understanding the language we refer to as *medical terminology.*

Medical terminology is defined as the use of specialized terms in the art and science of medicine. Considered a special language that originated with the ancient Greeks, it evolved as a result of the many advances in medicine throughout human history. As the scientific study of medicine and technology continued to advance, so too did the need to create universal words, symbols, and abbreviations that could be used by all medical practitioners throughout the world.

Most medical terms are composed of word parts and have their origins in ancient Greek or Latin. Because of this, it is necessary that the practitioner learn the English translation of terms when learning the fundamentals of word structures.

Fundamentals of Word Structure

The fundamental components found in medical terminology include four elements: the prefix, the root, the combining form, and the suffix.

Prefix. The term *prefix* pertains to attaching a syllable or group of syllables before, or to the beginning of, a word. It is used primarily either to alter or modify the meaning of the word or to create a new word.

For example, let's look at the word *antiseptic,* which pertains to an agent that works against sepsis. Note below how the components of the word are broken down:

Component	Meaning
anti (prefix)	away from
sept (root)	sepsis
ic (suffix)	pertaining to

Word root. A *root* is defined as a word or word element from which other words can be formed. It is the foundation of the word, conveying both a meaning and forming the base to which a prefix or suffix can be attached in order to modify the word.

For example, take the word *abnormal,* meaning to be away from the normal. Note below how we can break up the word into its component parts:

Component	Meaning
ab (prefix)	away from
norm (root)	rule
al (suffix)	pertaining to

Combining form. A *combining form* is defined as a word root to which a vowel has been affixed in order to join the root to a second root or to a suffix. The vowel *o* is used most often in the combining of words.

Look at the word *biology* below. It is defined as a term pertaining to the study of life.

Component	Meaning
bio (combining form)	pertaining to life
logy (suffix)	the study of

Suffix. A *suffix* is a word that means to "fasten beneath or under." It may be a syllable or a group of syllables united with or placed at the end of a word in order to alter or modify the meaning of the word, or to create a new word.

Look at the word *microscope* below. It is defined as an instrument used to view small objects.

Component	Meaning
micro (prefix)	*small*
scope (suffix)	*instrument to view*

Understanding Component Parts

Some medical terms have the same meanings as others. This generally occurs most often with words that relate to the organs of the body and the diseases that are affected by each. Usually this "double meaning" can be traced to differences in the Greek or Latin words from which these words originated. Most of the terms applied to the body's organs come from the Latin, whereas terms describing the diseases and disorders affecting the organs originate from the Greek.

For example, the term *uterus* is a Latin word that describes the organs of the female reproductive system, whereas the term *hyster,* a Greek root, describes the word for womb. Note that the commonly used prefixes listed below have more than a single meaning.

Prefix	Meaning
a, an	no, not, without, lack of, apart

Prefix	Meaning
ad	toward, near, to
dia	through, between
dys	bad, difficult, painful
ep, epi	upon, over, above
hypo	below, under, deficient
post	after, behind
supra	above, beyond

Now let's look at some of the more commonly used suffixes that have more than a single meaning:

Suffix	Meaning
blast	immature cell, germ cell
gram	weight, mark, record
penia	lack of, deficiency
rrhea	flow, discharge
scopy	to view, examine
stasis	control, stopping
trophy	nourishment, development
y	process, condition, pertaining to

Spelling

Medical terms that are of Greek origin are usually more difficult to spell because many of them begin with a silent letter or have a silent letter within the word. Look at the following examples.

Initial letter	Pronunciation	Example Medical Term
pn	"n"	pneumonia
ps	"s"	psychiatrist
pt	"t"	ptosis

Guidelines for Identification and Spelling of Medical Terms

Before we begin to study some of the more frequently used medical terms found in the study of electrocardiography, let's take a few moments to review some basic guidelines that will help in the identification and spelling of these terms:

1. If the suffix of a word begins with a vowel, always remember to drop the combining vowel from the combining form and add the suffix.

2. If the suffix of a word begins with a consonant, always remember to keep the combining vowel and add the suffix to the combining form.

3. Always keep the combining vowel between two or more roots in a term.

Forming Plural Endings

The term *plural* means more than one. To change a word from *singular,* pertaining to one, you will have to substitute the plural ending with a singular one. For example:

> *a* (singular) as in *bursa* becomes *ae* (plural) as in *bursae*
> *um* (singular) as in *ovum* become *a* (plural) as in *ova*

Pronounciation

At first, pronounciation of medical terms may seem difficult; however, it is very important to pronounce medical words with the same or very similar sounds in order to convey their correct meanings. Remember. . . just as in spelling, one mispronounced syllable can change the meaning of a medical word.

USING MEDICAL TERMINOLOGY RELATED TO ELECTROCARDIOGRAPHY

Now that you have a basic understanding of the principles involved in understanding the fundamental components of medical words, let's take a look at some of the more commonly used terms, abbreviations, and symbols used in the study of electrocardiography.

aneurysm: a spindle-shaped or saclike bulging of the wall of a vein or artery, usually due to a weakening of the wall by disease or an abnormality present at birth.

angina pectoris: literally, *chest pain;* a condition in which the heart muscle receives an insufficient blood supply, causing pain in the chest, and in some cases pain in the left arm and shoulder; commonly results when the arteries supplying the heart muscle (coronaries) become narrowed due to atherosclerosis.

angiocardiography: an X-ray examination of the heart and great blood vessels that follows the course of an opaque fluid that has been injected into the bloodstream.

anoxia: literally, *no oxygen;* a condition frequently occurring when the blood supply to a part of the body is completely cut off, with the result being death of the affected tissue.

anticoagulant: a drug that delays clotting of the blood; when given in cases of a clot in a blood vessel, anticoagulants tend to prevent new clots from forming or the existing clot from enlarging, but they do not dissolve the existing clot; examples include Heparin and Coumarin.

aorta: the main trunk artery that receives blood from the lower left chamber of the heart; responsible for supplying blood to all the lesser arteries that branch out through all parts of the body except the lungs.

aortic insufficiency: pertaining to an improper closing of the valve between the aorta and the lower-left chamber of the heart (left ventricle), which allows a back flow of blood.

aortic stenosis: a narrowing of the aortic valve either at the valve itself or slightly above or below the valve; may be the result of scar tissue forming after rheumatic fever, infarction, or may have other causes.

aortic valve: a valve located at the junction of the aorta and the lower-left chamber of the heart (left ventricle), formed by three cup-shaped membranes called *semilunar valves;* an aortic valve opens to allow blood to flow from the heart into the aorta and closes to prevent the back flow of this blood.

apex: the blunt, rounded end of the heart that is directed downward, forward, and to the left.

arrhythmia: an abnormal rhythm of the heart beat; a term generally used to describe all forms of abnormalities including disturbances in rate, rhythm and conduction in cardiac function.

arteriosclerosis: commonly referred to as "hardening of the arteries," a condition in which the walls of the arteries become thickened and hardened, loosing elasticity.

artery: blood vessels of systemic circulation that carry blood away from the heart to all parts of the body. (See Figure 2–1.)

atrio-ventricular node (A-V node):   a small mass of special muscle fibers at the base of the wall between the two upper chambers (atrium) of the heart; it forms the beginning of the bundle of His in the cardiac conduction system; the electrical impulse controlling the rhythm of the heart is initiated in the pacemaker cells of the S-A (sinoatrial) node, conducted through the muscle fibers of the right-upper chamber of the heart to the A-V node, and then conducted to the lower chambers of the heart by way of the bundle of His.

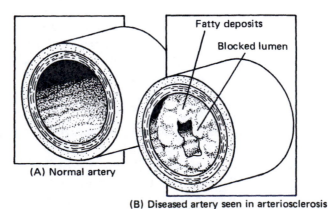

(A) Normal artery

(B) Diseased artery seen in arteriosclerosis

Figure 2–1   View of normal and diseased arteries.

atrium: one of the two upper chambers of the heart; also called the *auricle;* the right atrium receives oxygen-depleted blood from the body; the left atrium receives oxygen-rich blood from the lungs.

auricle: previously, the term for the upper chambers of the heart; generally used now to describe only the very tip of the atrium.

auscultation: the act of listening to sounds within the body, as in heart sounds.

bacterial endocarditis: an inflammation of the inner lining of the heart caused by bacteria; the lining of the heart valves are most commonly affected and can be a result of complications from an injury, surgery, or infectious diseases.

blood pressure: the pressure or force of blood in the arteries; composed of systolic blood pressure, pertaining to the heart muscle contracting, and diastolic blood pressure, seen when the heart muscle is relaxed between beats.

bradycardia: abnormally slow heart rate; generally any rate falling below 60 beats per minute is considered bradycardia.

bundle of His: a bundle of specialized muscle fibers originating in the A-V node; the bundle of His conducts the electrical impulse of cardiac conduction from the upper chambers of the heart (atria) to the lower chambers of the heart (ventricles); named after the German anatomist Wilhelm His.

cardiac: pertaining to the heart.

cardiac cycle: pertaining to one total heartbeat; one complete contraction and relaxation of the heart.

cardiac output: the amount of blood pumped by the heart per minute.

cardiopulmonary resuscitation (CPR): the act of performing both rescue breathing and chest compressions on a victim who has no respirations or pulse. (See Figure 2–2.)

cerebrovascular accident (CVA): sometimes called a *stroke,* a condition referring to an impeded blood supply to some part of the brain, generally caused by a blood clot, blood vessel rupture, partial clot from another part of the circulatory system, or pressure on the blood vessel, as in a tumor.

circulatory: pertaining to the heart, blood vessels, and the circulation of blood.

congestive heart failure: a condition in which the heart is unable adequately to pump out all the blood that returns to it, causing a backing up of blood in the veins leading to the heart.

coronary arteries: the two arteries, arising from the aorta, arching down over the top of the heart and conducting blood to the heart muscle.

cyanosis: blueness of the skin caused by a lack of insufficiency of oxygen in the blood.

defibrillator: any agent or procedure, such as an electric shock, which stops incoordinate contraction of the heart muscle and restores normal heart rhythm.

dyspnea: difficult or labored breathing.

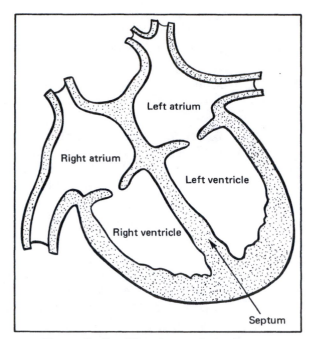

Figure 2-2   Chambers of the heart.

EKG/ECG: a graphic record of the electric currents produced by the heart.

edema: swelling due to abnormally large amounts of fluid accumulating in the tissues of the body.

electric cardiac pacemaker: an electric device that can control the beating of the heart by a rhythmic discharge of electrical impulses.

electrocardiograph: an instrument that records electric currents produced by the heart. (See Figure 2-3.)

embolism: the blocking of a blood vessel by a clot or other substance carried in the blood stream.

heart block: interference with the conduction of the electrical impulses of the heart which can be either partial or complete, and can result in dissociation of the rhythms of the upper and lower heart chambers.

hemiplegia: paralysis of one side of the body caused by a lack of blood and oxygen to the opposite side of the brain.

hemoglobin: the oxygen-carrying red pigment of the red blood cell (corpuscle); when it has absorbed oxygen in the lungs, it is bright red and is called *oxy-hemoglobin*; after it has given up its oxygen load in the tissues, it is purple in color and is called *reduced hemoglobin*.

heparin: a chemical substance that tends to prevent blood from clotting; an anticoagulant.

hypertension: commonly called *high blood pressure;* an unstable or persistent elevation of the blood pressure above the normal range, which may eventually lead to increased heart size and kidney damage.

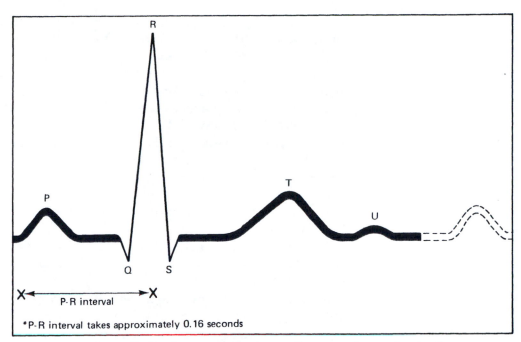

P-R interval

*P-R interval takes approximately 0.16 seconds

Figure 2–3   A normal electrocardiogram. Approximate time is 1 second from the beginning of the P-wave to the completion of the QRS-complex.

hypertrophy: the enlargement of a tissue or an organ due to increase in its size or bulk; may result from a demand in functional activity placed on the tissue or organ.

hypotension: commonly called *low blood pressure;* blood pressure falling below the normal range; most commonly used to describe an acute drop in blood pressure, as occurs in shock.

hypothermia: also called *hypothermy;* the lowering of the body temperature (usually to 86 to 88 degrees Fahrenheit), in order to slow the metabolic processes during heart surgery; in this cooled state, body tissues require less oxygen.

hypoxia: low oxygen content in the organs and tissues of the body.

incompetent valve: any valve that does not completely close and allows blood to leak back in the wrong direction; also called *valvular insufficiency.*

infarct (infarction):   an area of tissue damaged or dead as a result of an insufficient blood supply; myocardial infarct (infarction) refers to an area of the heart muscle damaged or killed by an insufficient flow of blood through the coronary arteries that normally supply it.

insufficiency: incompetency; in the condition termed *valvular insufficiency,* an improper closing of the valves, which admits a back flow of blood in the wrong direction; in the condition termed *myocardial insufficiency,* pertains to an inability of the heart muscle to function normally as a pump for circulation.

interatrial septum: sometimes called *atrial septum;* a muscular wall dividing the left and right upper chambers of the heart.

interventricular septum: also called the *ventricular septum;* the muscular wall dividing the left and right lower chambers of the heart.

ischemia: a local, usually temporary, deficiency of blood in some area of the body, often caused by a constriction or an obstruction in the blood vessel supplying that part.

jugular veins: veins that return blood from the head and neck to the heart.

mitral stenosis: a narrowing of the valve (called the *bicuspid* or *mitral valve*) opening between the upper and lower chamber in the left side of the heart; sometimes the result of scar tissue forming after rheumatic fever infection.

mitral valve: also called the *bicuspid valve;* consists of two cups of triangular segments, located between the upper and lower chambers of the left side of the heart.

murmur: an abnormal heart sound heard between the normal "lub-dub" heart sounds.

myocardial infarction: damage or death of an area of heart muscle (myocardium) resulting from a reduction in the blood supply to that area.

myocardial insufficiency: inability of the heart muscle to maintain normal circulation.

myocarditis: inflammation of the heart muscle (myocardium).

myocardium: the muscular wall of the heart; the thickest of the three layers of the heart wall, it lies between the inner layer (endocardium) and the outer layer (epicardium). (See Figure 2–4.)

palpitation: fluttering of the heart; abnormal rate or rhythm of the heartbeat.

paroxysmal tachycardia: a period of rapid heartbeats that begins and ends suddenly.

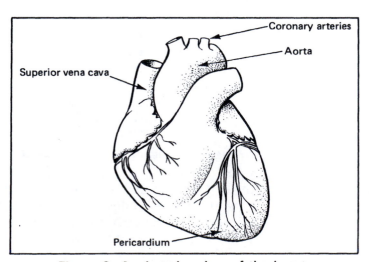

Figure 2–4 Anterior view of the heart.

pulse: the expansion and contraction of an artery that may be felt by placing the fingers on the artery.

stasis: a stoppage or slackening of the blood flow.

symptom: any sign or indication of the patient's condition.

syncope: fainting.

tachycardia: abnormally rapid heart rate, generally anything over 100 beats per minute.

thrombosis: the formation or presence of a blood clot (thrombus) inside a blood vessel or cavity of the heart.

tricuspid valve: a valve consisting of three cusps or triangular segments located between the upper and lower chamber of the right side of the heart; its position corresponds to the bicuspid, or mitral valve, on the left side of the heart.

vagus nerves: nerves of the parasympathetic nervous system that extend from the brain and slow the heart rate when stimulated.

vasoconstrictor: nerves or chemical agents that cause vessels to relax, thus increasing the flow of blood and the lowering of blood pressure.

vein: any one of a series of vessels of the vascular system that carries blood from the various parts of the body back to the heart; all veins in the body carry unoxygenated blood, except the pulmonary veins.

vena cava: the main vein returning blood from the body to the right atrium.

ventricle: one of the two lower chambers of the heart; left ventricle pumps oxygenated blood through the arteries to the body in systemic circulation; right ventricle pumps blood through the pulmonary arteries to the lungs in pulmonary circulation.

ventricular septum: sometimes called the *interventricular* septum; it is the muscular wall that divides the two lower chambers of the heart.

EKG SYMBOLS AND ABBREVIATIONS

The following is a list of symbols and abbreviations most commonly used in the study of electrocardiography.

QID	four times a day	**DC**	discontinue; discharge
TID	three times a day	**BP**	blood pressure
QH	every hour	**TPR**	temperature, pulse, respiration
BID	twice a day		
Stat	immediately	**SOB**	short of breath
QD	everyday		
$\overline{\text{c}}$	with	**CVA**	cerebrovascular accident (stroke)
$\overline{\text{s}}$	without		
$\overline{\text{p}}$	after		

PRN	whenever necessary	**Wt**	weight
cc	cubic centimeter	**LLQ**	left lower quadrant
CCU	coronary care unit	**LUQ**	left upper quadrant
EKG	electrocardiogram	**GI**	gastrointestinal
Fx	fracture	**Dr.**	doctor
AM	morning	**>**	greater than
ER	emergency room	**<**	less than
H&P	history and physical	**A-V node**	atrioventricular node
IV	intravenous	**S-A node**	sinoatrial node
NPO	nothing by mouth (Latin: *nil per os*)	**MI**	myocardial infarction
CATH	catheterization; as in cardiac catheterization	**AC interference**	alternating current interference; pertaining to the EKG tracing
Dx	diagnosis	**NSR**	normal sinus rhythm
Trt	treatment		
Sympt	symptom	**megaly**	enlarged
Pt	patient	**micro**	small; tiny; microscopic
PM	afternoon		
Post-op	after surgery	**scopy**	to view
Pre-op	before surgery	**pnea**	pertaining to breathing
NG	nasogastric		
R	respiration	**hypo**	below; decreased
®	rectal		
O₂	oxygen	**hyper**	above; increased
Rx	pertaining to dispensing of medication	**QNS**	quantity not sufficient
DOA	dead on arrival	**QS**	quantity sufficient
CHF	congestive heart failure	**RLQ**	right lower quadrant
CNS	central nervous system	**RUQ**	right upper quadrant
e.g.	as in	**Amb**	ambulate
L	liter	**URI**	upper respiratory infection
Ht	height		

P	pulse	**glyco**	sugar
pre	pertaining to before	**necro**	death
		pathy	condition of
post	pertaining to after	**COPD**	chronic obstructive pulmonary disease
semi	half		
hemi	half		
hema	blood		

Medical Abbreviations Related to Time

a.c.	before meals	**b.i.d.**	twice a day
p.c.	after meals	**t.i.d.**	three times a day
AM	morning	**q.i.d.**	four times a day
PM	afternoon or evening	**q.2h**	every 2 hours
		q.4h	every 4 hours
h.s.	hour of sleep (bedtime)	**q.12h**	every 12 hours
hr	hour		

Medical Abbreviations Related to Places or Departments

OR	operating room	**EENT**	eye, ear, nose, and throat
Lab	laboratory		
ICU	intensive care unit	**GI**	gastrointestinal
OPD	outpatient department	**ER**	emergency room
		CS	central supply
CCU	coronary care unit	**Gyn**	gynecology
OB	obstetrics	**Peds**	pediatrics

Medical Abbreviations Related to Patient Orders

ADL	activities of daily living	**s̄**	without
prn	whenever necessary	**gtt.**	drops
		lb.	pound
stat	immediately	**wt.**	weight
ad. lib.	as desired	**ht.**	height
dc	discontinue	**NPO**	nothing by mouth
spec.	specimen	**p.o.**	by mouth
O₂	oxygen	**per**	by
tinct.	tincture	**liq.**	liquid
q.s.	quantity sufficient	**B.M.**	bowel movement
Q	every	**P.O.**	post-operative
ung.	ointment	**preop**	pre-operative
s̄s̄	one-half	**pt**	pint (500 ml)
c̄	with	**L**	liter (1,000 ml, quart)

Medical Abbreviations Related to Patient Orders (cont)

amt	amount	**Dr**	doctor
Rx	treatment (take)	**Dx**	diagnosis

Medical Abbreviations Related to History and Physical

CHF	congestive heart failure	**CVA**	cerebrovascular accident (stroke)
RHD	rheumatic heart disease	**URI**	upper respiratory infection
ASHD	arteriosclerotic heart disease	**PID**	pelvic inflammatory disease
CO	coronary occlusion	**MS**	multiple sclerosis
MI	myocardial infarction	**STD**	sexually transmitted disease

Roman Numerals

I	1	VI	6	XX	20
II	2	VII	7	L	50
III	3	VIII	8	C	100
IV	4	IX	9	M	1,000
V	5	X	10		

Abbreviations Related to Measurements and Volume

oz	ounce	**cc**	cubic centimeter
dr	dram	**ml**	milliliter
c	centimeter	**L**	liter

Abbreviations Related to Height and Weight

lb	pounds
in	inches
kg	kilogram

Abbreviations Related to Temperature

F	Fahrenheit
C	celsius or centigrade
°	degree

COMMONLY USED PREFIXES

Prefix	Meaning	Prefix	Meaning
a, an	without; lack of	*arthro*	joint
ab	away from	*ad*	toward

Prefix	Meaning	Prefix	Meaning
adeno	gland	*hepato*	liver
amnio	sack	*histo*	tissue
angi	vessel	*hydro*	water
angio	vessel	*hyper*	excessive; above
ante	before	*hypo*	under; below
anti	against	*icter*	yellow
antr	chamber	*inter*	between
apo	detached	*intra*	within; inside
athero	fattylike tissue	*leuko*	white
auto	self	*lipo*	fat
axilla	armpit	*litho*	stone
bi	two	*mal*	bad; abnormal
bio	life	*mammo*	breast
blast	developing	*masto*	breast
brady	slow	*melano*	black
cap	head	*morpho*	shape; form
carcin	cancer	*myo*	muscle
cardio	heart	*neo*	new
cervico	neck	*nephro*	kidney
chole	gallbladder	*neuro*	nerve
colo	large intestine	*oligo*	small amount
contra	against	*oophoro*	ovary
craneo	skull	*op; ophth*	eye; vision
cyst	sac	*optic*	eye; vision
chloro	green	*orchi*	testicle
cyan	blue	*orth*	straight
cyto	cell	*osteo*	bone
derm	skin	*oto; auri*	ear
dia	across	*para*	beside; near
diplo	double	*pedi*	child
dis	apart	*peri*	around
dys	bad or painful	*phleb (o)*	vein
enceph	brain	*phobia*	fear
endo	inside	*physio*	nature
epi	union or after	*pleuro*	membrane lung
erythro	red	*pneumo*	lung
exo	outside	*poly*	many; much
gastro	stomach	*procto*	rectum
hema	blood	*pseudo*	false
hemo	blood	*psyche*	mind

COMMONLY USED SUFFIXES

Suffix	Meaning	Suffix	Meaning
algia	pain	oma	tumor
centesis	surgical puncture	osis	condition of
cyte	cell	ostomy	a new opening
ectomy	removal of	penia	decrease
emia	condition of the blood	plasty	repair
gram	picture; recording	ptosis	falling
graph	picture, recording	rrhagia	breaking
itis	inflammation	rrhaphy	suture; sew
ist	specialist	scope	instrument for viewing
megaly	enlargement	stasis	control, stopping
natal	birth	trophy	nourishment, development
oid	resembling	uria	urine
ology	study of		
orrhea	flow; discharge		

ABBREVIATIONS RELATED TO MEDICATIONS

Abbreviation	Meaning	Abbreviation	Meaning
aa	of each	Gm	gram
a.c.	before meals	gr	grain
ad	to	gtt	drop
ad lib	as desired	H; hypo	hypodermic
amp	ampule	h	hour
aq	water	hs	hour of sleep
aq dist	distilled water	IM	intramuscular
bid	twice a day	IV	intravenous
bin	twice a night	L	liter
cap	capsule	liq	liquid
$\bar{c}$	with	m	minim
cc	cubic centimeter	mg	milligram
comp	compound	mEq	milli-equivalent
DC	discontinue	noc; n	night
dr	dram	non rep	no repeat
elix	elixir	ol	oil
EC	enteric coated	OD	right eye
ext	extract	OU	both eyes
Fe	iron	OS	left eye
Fld	fluid		

REVIEW QUESTIONS

Directions: For each section below, give the answers you believe are most correct:

1. Match the terms in Column A by entering the correct number of the definition (Column B) in the space provided:

Column A

_____ angina pectoris

_____ circulatory

_____ thrombosis

_____ cardiac cycle

_____ hypertension

_____ palpitation

_____ infarct

_____ arrhythmia

_____ stasis

_____ insufficiency

_____ tachycardia

_____ cerebrovascular accident

_____ paroxysmal tachycardia

_____ symptom

_____ bradycardia

_____ pulse

_____ syncope

_____ anoxia

_____ cardiac output

Column B

1. without oxygen
2. amount of blood pumped by heart per minute
3. expansion and contraction of an artery, felt by placing fingers on the artery
4. abnormally high blood pressure
5. pain in chest due to spasm
6. one complete heartbeat
7. pertaining to heart, blood vessels, and circulation of blood
8. difficult or labored breathing
9. stoppage of blood flow
10. formation or presence of blood clot inside a blood vessel or cavity of the heart
11. any sign or indication of the patient's condition
12. abnormal rhythm of heartbeat
13. sometimes called a stroke
14. incompetency
15. abnormally slow heartbeat
16. area of tissue damaged as a result of insufficient blood supply
17. blueness of skin caused by insufficient oxygen in blood
18. fainting
19. fluttering of the heart; abnormal rate or rhythm of beat
20. abnormally rapid heart rate; generally anything over 100 beats per minute
21. a period of rapid heart beats that begins and ends suddenly

2. Match the following abbreviations by putting the correct letter in the space provided:

_____ QID	A. with
_____ Qh	B. immediately
_____ STAT	C. greater than
_____ c̄	D. temperature, pulse, respiration
_____ BID	E. four times a day
_____ DC	F. short of breath
_____ p̄	G. less than
_____ >	H. three times a day
_____ <	I. discontinue
_____ TPR	J. cerebrovascular accident
_____ TID	K. after
_____ QD	L. every day
_____ s̄	M. without
_____ SOB	N. twice a day
_____ BP	O. blood pressure
_____ CVA	P. every hour

3. Define the following abbreviations related to places or departments:

(a) OR _____

(b) ICU _____

(c) CCU _____

(d) ER _____

(e) CS _____

(f) PEDS _____

(g) OB _____

(h) LAB _____

(i) OPD _____

(j) EENT _____

4. Define the following abbreviations related to patient orders:

(a) gtt _____

(b) NPO _____

(c) ad lib _____

(d) prn _____

(e) q.s. _____

(f) ADL _____

(g) O$_2$ _____

(h) Spec _____

(i) Rx _____

(j) Dx _____

5. Give the Arabic number for the following Roman numerals:

(a) VI _____   (f) CCC _____

(b) VII _____   (g) M _____

(c) VIII _____   (h) XXXV _____

(d) IX _____   (i) XIX _____

(e) X _____   (j) CXXV _____

6. Define the following prefixes:

(a) arthro _____

(b) athero _____

(c) auto _____

(d) ad _____

(e) anti _____

(f) ante _____

(g) cardio _____

(h) hema _____

(i) para _____

(j) intra _____

7. Define the following suffixes:

   (a) algia _____

   (b) graph _____

   (c) itis _____

   (d) rrhagia _____

   (e) megaly _____

   (f) orrhea _____

   (g) plasty _____

   (h) trophy _____

   (i) ostomy _____

   (j) stasis _____

8. Define the following abbreviations related to medications:

   (a) a.c. _____

   (b) a.q. _____

   (c) Gm _____

   (d) gr _____

   (e) hs _____

   (f) IM _____

   (g) L _____

   (h) OD _____

   (i) mg _____

   (j) Fe _____

Anatomy and Physiology
of the Heart
and Cardiovascular System

3

TERMINAL OBJECTIVE

To provide the student with a brief overview of the anatomy and physiology of the heart and the cardiovascular system and their relationship to the process and techniques involved in the performance of recording an electrocardiogram.

COMPETENCY OBJECTIVES

Upon completion of this chapter, the student will be able to

1. Correctly spell and define terminology related to the study of anatomy and physiology of the heart and the cardiovascular system.
2. Describe the normal position of the heart and its valves.
3. Describe the gross structure and function of the pericardium, chambers, and muscle cells of the heart.
4. Describe the innervation, blood flow, and blood supply of the heart.
5. Discuss the conduction system of the heart.
6. Explain the process of the cardiac cycle of the heart.

ANATOMY OF THE HEART

The human heart is an organ approximately the size of a man's fist. It is a hollow muscle divided into four chambers, and its main function is to pump blood. It is located in the *mediastinum,* or the middle section of the thorax, or chest, between the lungs, with its apex, or pointed end, resting on the diaphragm.

Each heart chamber is separated by heart valves, which act as gatelike structures, opening in only one direction. This keeps the blood flowing one way, thereby preventing it from "backing up." When the heart beats or contracts, two of the valves, the *tricuspid* and the *mitral,* close. When the heart relaxes, the other two valves, the *aortic* and the *pulmonary,* close. When a valve closes, it makes a sound. This is the characteristic "lub-dub" that is heard by an instrument known as a stethoscope when the valves close.

The actual anatomical location of the four cardiac valves to the anterior, or front, of the thoracic wall is different from the clinical valvular areas that can be examined by *auscultation,* or the process of listening to sounds of the body. The reason for this difference is the actual location of the heart valves, with respect to the chest, and the correct location for placing the stethoscope. And it is due to any physical problems that may be concerned with the production and conduction of the heart sound, since sound travels along tissue and not necessarily straight through the chest wall. (See Figure 3–1.)

Heart Sounds

As we have already stated, there are two main heart sounds that can be heard under normal conditions and that are responsible for making the classic "lub-dub" sound. The first sound, or the "lub," is the louder of the two and is associated with the closing of the tricuspid and mitral valves. The second sound, or the "dub," is made as a result of the closing of the aortic and pulmonary valves.

The Heart Chambers

We already know that the heart is a muscular organ, about the size of a man's fist. If we were to cut open this organ we would see it has four chambers, the right atrium, the right ventricle, the left atrium, and the left ventricle.

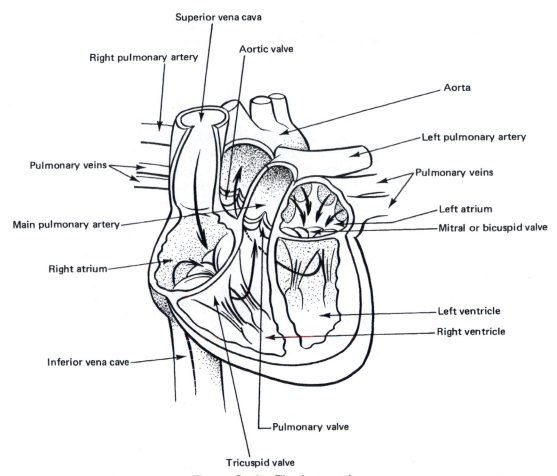

Figure 3-1   The human heart at rest.

The Pericardium

The heart is contained within a sac called the *pericardium*. This sac is filled with a pericardial fluid, which moistens the lining of the pericardium and the epicardium, or outer surface of the heart.

Normally, there is approximately 10 to 20cc of thin, clear pericardial fluid that moistens the contracting surfaces of the epicardium and the inner surface of the pericardium.

The Septum, Ventricles, and Atrium

The four chambers of the heart are separated by a structure called the *septum*, or muscle wall. The two lower chambers, called the *ventricles*, are responsible for pumping blood away from the heart, while the two upper chambers, the *atrium*, are responsible for receiving the blood coming to the heart. The valves, which we have already discussed, are the structures that maintain the control of the blood flowing through the entire heart.

The left ventricle does more work than does the right ventricle and, as a result, has the thickest wall. It is responsible for pumping oxygenated blood to all parts of the body, except for the lungs, and eventually empties its blood directly into the aorta. Because the left ventricle pumps blood a very long way, it is referred to as a *high-pressure pump.*

Blood enters the right atrium from all parts of the body and empties into the right ventricle via the tricuspid valve. The right ventricle pumps the nonoxygenated blood to the lungs via the pulmonary artery. The right ventricle is considered a *low-pressure pump* and therefore has a thinner wall than does the left ventricle.

The interventricular septum is also a thick wall that is responsible for separating the left and right ventricles. This wall will constrict during a heartbeat in order to provide a rigid structure during the heart contraction. If this did not occur, the high pressure that develops in the left ventricle during the contraction would cause a thin septum to bulge into the low-pressure right ventricle and eventually would interfere with its operation.

The action occurring within the atrium has to do with two main functions. Considered the receiving chambers of the heart, the left atrium is responsible for receiving the oxygenated blood from the lungs via the pulmonary veins, while the right atrium receives the nonoxygenated blood from the rest of the body. The superior vena cava and the inferior vena cava are the two great veins that enter into the right atrium.

The Heart Valves

As we have previously indicated, the heart valves have the major responsibility of preventing blood from backing up as it flows through the heart. There are two types of valves found in the heart—the *atrioventricular* valves, such as the tricuspid and the mitral valves, and the *semilunar,* such as the pulmonary and aortic valves. All heart valves are mechanical structures, and they are constructed in such a way as to permit the blood to flow only one direction within the circulatory system.

The Atrioventricular Valves

The atrioventricular valves, which include the bicuspid, or mitral, and the tricuspid, are thin structures located between the atrium and the ventricles.

The tricuspid valve, located at the right atrioventricular opening, got its name because of its structure, consisting of three "cusps," or flaps. These cusps are continuous with each other at their bases, thereby forming a ring-shaped membrane, which surround the arterial passage of blood.

The left atrioventricular opening is guarded by the bicuspid or mitral valve and derives its name from its two cusps, or flaps. Its attachment is the same as for the tricuspid valve, except that it is much thicker, thereby corresponding to the thicker wall of the left ventricle, an occurrence made necessary by the heavy pumping load undertaken by the left ventricle.

When the atrioventricular valves are open, blood is then able to pass freely from the atrium to the ventricles, as the atrium contracts. Filling the ventricles with blood from the contracting atrium then causes the atrioventricular valves to close and thereby prevents the backflow of blood into the atrium when the ventricles contract.

The semilunar valves differ in their function from the atrioventricular valves, primarily because of their shape. Looking very much like a half-moon, they come out from the lining of the pulmonary artery and the aorta. The major responsibility of the semilunar valves is to prevent any blood from flowing back into the ventricles as it makes its way from the pulmonary artery and the aorta.

TRACING THE FLOW OF BLOOD THROUGH THE HEART

Now that you understand the basic structure of the chambers and valves located within the heart, it is important for you to note how the blood makes its way through this organ.

To begin with, the right atrium receives the blood. It then moves through the tricuspid valve to the right ventricle, through the pulmonary semilunar valve and into the lungs, and back through the left atrium. Once the blood leaves the left atrium, it flows through the bicuspid, or mitral valve, into the left ventricle, through the aortic semilunar valve, and eventually out to the rest of the body.

CARDIAC MUSCLE CELLS

When learning about the anatomy and physiology of the heart, and how it relates to the electrical activity occurring during the heart's contraction and relaxation phases, it is also important that you understand how the cells of the cardiac muscles play a major role in the heart's activity.

The cells are most concerned with the mechanical activity of the heart; therefore, they are all similar in their appearance. This applies to both the atrial and the ventricular cells. The principal function of all cardiac muscle cells is to contract. Because of the cell's shape—that is, rectangular, with an oval-shaped nucleus—it also interconnects with neighboring cells.

The cardiac muscle cells make up three major layers, or portions, of the heart. The inner layer, which is responsible for lining the chambers of the heart, is called the *endocardium.* Its thin, shiny, smooth membrane also lines or covers the heart valves and is therefore continuous with the lining of the large blood vessels.

The outer layer of the heart is called the *epicardium,* which is made up of thick muscular cells, while the middle layer, called the *myocardium,* is constructed of interlacing cardiac muscle fibers. Because of the consistency of the muscle fibers comprising the myocardium, this is the layer responsible for causing the heart to contract.

BLOOD VESSELS AND CIRCULATION

Whenever we discuss the anatomy and physiology of the heart and the cardiovascular system, it is also important to spend some time talking about the blood vessels—that is, those structures that assist the body in its circulation of blood and other important body fluids.

Although there are many different types, sizes, and varieties of blood vessels contained within the human body, all of them may be classified into three major groups: *arteries,* which are responsible for carrying oxygenated blood away from the heart; *veins,* which carry nonoxygenated blood toward the heart; and *capillaries,* which are tiny, microscopic structures most responsible for allowing the rapid exchange of substances between the blood and the tissue cells.

Arteries

As we have already stated, arteries are blood vessels most responsible for carrying oxygenated blood away from the heart, with the one exception being the pulmonary artery. The largest of all arteries in the human body is called the *aorta,* which measures approximately 25 mm, and is about one inch in diameter. As other arteries branch off the aorta, they become smaller and smaller, until they reach the tissue level, at which time they become *arterioles,* which are approximately 30 microns in diameter (a micron is 0.001 mm).

All arteries consist of three layers of tissue: the *tunica adventitia,* which is the outer layer, consisting of tough, fibrous connective tissue; the *tunica media,* or the middle layer, composed of smooth muscle, white fibrous and elastic tissue, which permits the vessel to dilate and constrict; and the *tunica intima,* or the inner layer, which consists of a layer of endothelial cells. (See Figure 3–2.)

Veins

Veins, unlike arteries, are most concerned with carrying the nonoxygenated blood from the capillaries toward the heart. Although consisting of the same three layers as found in the arteries, in veins the layers are much thinner and contain fewer elastic fibers. In contrast to the walls of the arteries, which if cut will remain open, the walls of the veins, once cut, will then collapse. (See Figure 3–3.)

Capillaries

Considered the one structure most responsible for the rapid exchange of substances between the blood and the tissue cells, capillaries are defined as tiny, microscopic vessels composed of a single layer of endothelial cells.

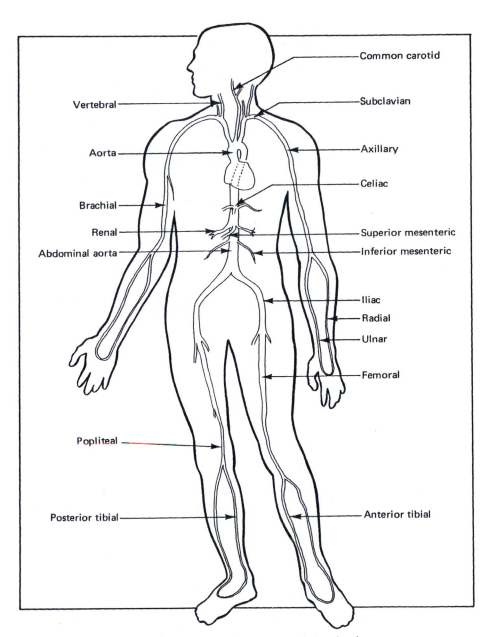

Figure 3-2 Major arteries of the body.

Capillaries function at the cellular level; they transport and diffuse essential materials to and from the body's cells and the blood.

UNDERSTANDING CIRCULATION

Now that we have discussed the three structures most responsible for the circulation of blood and other body fluids, let's take a look at the role each plays in this function.

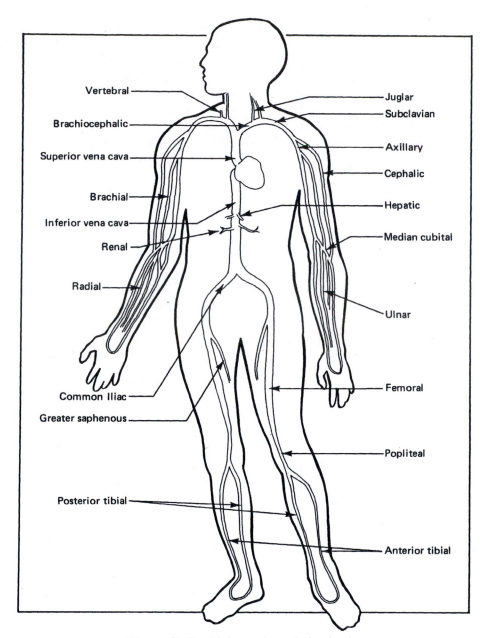

Figure 3-3 Major veins of the body.

It is important that you first understand that there are two main methods, or systems, involved in the circulation of the blood and other fluids within the body. They are the pulmonary system and the systemic system.

Pulmonary circulation includes all the blood vessels to and from the lungs, with the one exception being the bronchiolar arteries, which are responsible for supplying oxygenated blood to the lung tissue. During pulmonary circulation, the pulmonary artery delivers blood from the heart to the lungs, while the pulmonary veins deliver the blood from the lungs to the left atrium of the heart. The pulmonary circulation is different from systemic circulation in that it is a low-pressure system and has only vessels in which an artery, the pulmonary artery, carries nonoxygenated blood, whereas the veins carry oxygenated blood.

The systemic system differs from pulmonary circulation in that it includes all other blood vessels, beginning with the aorta, which eventually branches into smaller arteries, and finally arterioles. The system also includes microscopic capillary exchange vessels as well as venules, which are microscopic veins responsible for collecting returning nonoxygenated blood from the capillaries, which eventually empty into the veins, when transporting nonoxygenated blood to the vena cava and finally to the right atrium.

VEINS AND THE LYMPH SYSTEM

As previously noted, veins are thin-walled vessels responsible for returning nonoxygenated blood to the right atrium. These vessels have small valves spaced intermittently along their length that prevent any backflow of blood. The muscles of the body that surround the veins put pressure on them during normal movements of the body, thereby helping to force venous blood to the heart. Blood is also forced through the capillaries by the heart.

The Lymphatic System

Blood is responsible not only for supplying the cells of the body with food and oxygen but also for removing waste products. This exchange takes place at the capillary level. In addition, the tissue fluid that bathes the cells and therefore acts as a connecting link between the blood and the cells is called *lymph.* Lymph is formed when certain parts of the blood plasma pass through the capillary walls into the tissue spaces and is continually being drained from the tissue spaces through a system of tubules called the *lymphatic system.*

The lymphatic network begins as tiny lymph capillaries, which are somewhat similar to the blood capillaries. These vessels eventually become larger lymphatic vessels that parallel the veins. The lymphatic vessels eventually converge and empty into the lymphatic ducts.

Two major ducts are present in the lymphatic system. The first, called the *lymphatic duct,* is responsible for draining lymph from the head, neck, and right chest. The second major duct is called the *thoracic duct.* It is responsible for draining lymph from the remainder of the body. Once both ducts have completed their respective tasks, each empties lymph into both the right and left jugular veins.

All lymphatic vessels house tiny lymph glands or nodes, which are small structures located at key points along the side of the vessel. They are most dense in the axilla, or armpit, and the groin region of the body.

The flow of lymph is aided by small valves that are similar to the valves found in the veins. These valves prevent the backflow of lymph.

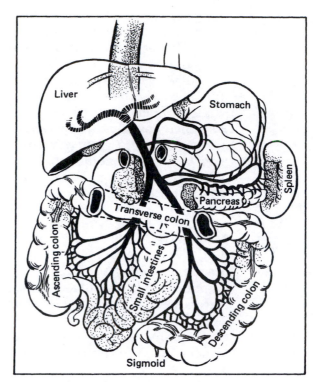

Figure 3-4   The portal system.

The lymph flow is also aided by pressure gradient between high tissue pressure and low lymphatic duct pressure.

It is important to note that the lymphatic system is the only means by which protein, or albumin, may leave the vascular compartment to be returned back to the blood. This is because protein diffusion, or breakup, may not occur within the capillaries. If this protein were not removed by the lymph, it would then accumulate in the tissue space and eventually produce edema, or swelling. In addition to protein drainage, the lymphatic nodes also filter the lymph and remove any foreign particles, such as bacteria. The lymph nodes also add a rich supply of lymphocytes, or white blood cells, to the lymph, which in turn transports these cells into the venous blood. (See Figure 3-4.)

CORONARY CIRCULATION

The term *coronary circulation* pertains to the flow of blood that takes place throughout the coronary arteries located in the heart. These arteries are responsible for carrying oxygenated blood to the heart muscle itself. This blood supply is then carried off of the aorta, which is the largest artery found in the heart and located just above the aortic valves.

There is both a left and right main coronary artery. The left coronary artery branches into two coronary arteries—the left anterior descending and the left circumflex branches. The right coronary artery is located on the posterior, or back side, and to the right of the heart.

After the oxygenated blood is carried to the myocardial tissue by the coronary arteries, the oxygen is then exchanged for carbon dioxide and the returning nonoxygenated blood is returned by the coronary veins, which are responsible for emptying into the coronary sinus. This in turn empties into the right atrium.

Because the heart requires a constant supply of oxygenated blood in order to provide sufficient oxygen to maintain energy for a constantly beating heart, the function of the coronary arteries is to provide the heart with the oxygenated blood. If the arterial supply is cut off, the heart will suffer a lack of oxygen, resulting in what is referred to as a *myocardial infarction*, or heart attack, caused by the death of the heart tissue. Therefore, the maintenance of coronary arterial blood is vital to sustaining life.

Flow of Blood Through the Heart

The flow of blood through the heart follows a very specific direction. It begins with the left ventricle pumping oxygenated blood to the aorta, which then carries blood to the systemic arteries. These arteries, in turn, supply all of the tissues of the body, with the exception of the lungs.

The nonoxygenated blood returning from the tissues is then carried by veins and returns to the heart through the superior and inferior vena cava. The nonoxygenated blood of the vena cava enters the right atrium and then flows into the right ventricle. The right ventricle pumps the nonoxygenated blood into the pulmonary artery, which carries it into the lungs.

After the lungs have exchanged oxygen for carbon dioxide, the newly oxygenated blood returns from the lung through the pulmonary veins, which in turn empty the oxygenated blood into the left atrium, eventually completing the emptying process into the left ventricle.

INNERVATION, BLOOD FLOW, AND BLOOD SUPPLY

The heart is responsible for receiving nerve fibers from the sympathetic nerves, which in turn eventually terminate upon the sinoatrial node (SA node) and atrioventricular node (AV node). In addition, because these nerves also terminate at the myocardium, or middle layer of the heart, the heart also receives a certain amount of blood flowing from the parasympathetic nerves. Like the sympathetic nerves, the parasympathetic also terminate at the SA and AV nodes.

All cardiac muscle cells have an inherent, or characteristic, rate of contraction called *depolarization*. What this means is that the heart maintains a beat unless other stimuli are received. The sympathetic and parasympathetic nerves can therefore influence the heartbeat rate, but in opposite directions.

Parasympathetic nerves also have the capacity to cause the heart rate to decrease, while the sympathetic nerves have the opposite influence—that is, they may cause the heart rate to increase. The two have the dual responsibility of working together in order to balance the heart rate and thereby maintain a normal heart rate, usually between 60 to 100 beats per minute for an average healthy adult.

During exercise, or any other strenuous activity, the heart rate increases because of the sympathetic nerve activity. In addition to affecting the heart's rate, these nerves may also cause the heart to contract with greater force, while the parasympathetic nerves have no influence on the strength of the heart's contractions.

UNDERSTANDING THE CARDIAC CYCLE

As previously stated, the normal, healthy heart beats approximately 60 to 100 times per minute, and this number of beats per minute is referred to as the *heart rate,* which is reflected in what we call the *cardiac cycle.* While there are a number of events that take place during a cardiac cycle, the most important point to remember is that the cardiac cycle is the time which is created from one heartbeat to the next; the time when the cardiac muscle contracts, forcing the blood to move out through the arteries, and eventually causing the muscles of the ventricles to relax. In essence, what occurs during the cardiac cycle is both a muscular contraction and a muscular relaxation. At the end of the contraction, the muscles begin to relax, thereby causing the incoming arterial blood to expand the muscle fibers and the relaxed muscle fibers to lengthen. Within normal limits, the longer the muscle fibers lengthen, the greater will be the contraction.

When the myocardium completes its contraction, it is referred to as *systole.* Then, as the myocardium begins to relax, it becomes dilated by the inrushing atrial blood. This is called *diastole.* Both the atrial and the ventricular myocardium exhibit systole and diastole, and the cardiac cycle cannot be complete until the atrium finishes its contraction before the ventricles begin their phase.

Blood Pressure and the Cardiac Cycle

The term *blood pressure* pertains to the time spent during the heart's contraction and relaxation. Systole, as we have already mentioned, not only occurs during the time spent when the myocardium completes its contraction, but also is defined as the maximum pressure formed during a ventricular contraction. Diastole, on the other hand, is not only created by an inrushing of atrial blood, as the myocardium begins to relax, but it is also defined as the minimum pressure during the ventricular relaxation phase.

When measured, blood pressure is determined and recorded in millimeters of mercury (mmHg). Thus, in a blood pressure of 120/80, the 120 represents the systolic pressure, or the time in which the heart is contracting, and the 80 represents the diastolic pressure, or the time in which the heart is relaxing.

UNDERSTANDING THE CONDUCTION SYSTEM OF THE HEART

The heart, as we have already stated, acts very much like a pump, actually "pumping" blood from its origination point to all parts of the body. During this pumping action, electrical impulses are also being created by certain anatomical structures located within the heart itself. It is these electrical impulses that are measured during the electrocardiogram ordered by the physician.

The structures creating the electrical impulses or stimuli make up the *conduction system.* They include the sinoatrial, or SA node; the atrioventricular, or AV node; the bundle of His; and the Purkinje fibers.

The SA Node

The sinoatrial, or SA node, located in the right atrium at the opening of the superior vena cava into the right atrium, is made up of a group of cells responsible for generating electrical impulses spontaneously and repeatedly. It is for this reason that it is most commonly referred to as the "pacemaker" of the heart. It is stimulated by both sympathetic and parasympathetic nerves, which in turn regulate the heart rate.

The cells of the SA node have the ability to generate a small electrical charge, which in a normal, healthy person fire off in short, rhythmic bursts, much like the flashing of an automobile turn signal. Each short burst of electrical current then depolarizes the muscle cells, causing the atrial muscle to contract. As the electrical current begins to cause the atrial muscle to contract, it also spreads along each muscle fiber toward the AV node.

The AV Node

Located in the right atrial muscle tissue at the junction of the atrium and the intraventricular septum, the AV, or atrioventricular, node is most responsible for receiving parasympathetic and sympathetic nerve fibers. As the electrical current is generated and spread from the SA node, it causes the AV node to "fire off." Once the AV node picks up the electrical charge, it then is responsible for relaying the current to the *bundle of His.*

The Bundle of His

Consisting of both a right and left branch, the bundle of His is located in the intraventricular septum near the base of the heart. Alongside each of the branches, the AV bundles give off small fibers that project into the ventricular muscle fibers. Once the electrical charge has been sent from the AV node to the bundle of His, it is then relayed into each AV bundle. Finally, the electrical current spreads from the AV bundle into the small fibers, called *Purkinje fibers,* eventually causing the cardiac muscles to contract. It is important to note that the electrical stimulus that has been conducted from the SA node all the way to the muscle fiber occurs very rapidly, in actuality in hundredths of a second.

Sequence of Events During the Conduction Phase

As we have already stated, the instrument used to measure the electrical impulses of the heart is called an electrocardiograph machine. During this measurement, while the heart is contracting and relaxing, certain events are taking place in the heart that cause these electrical impulses to occur.

During the heart's conduction, the SA node is first activated, followed by atrial contraction. This is followed by the AV node being activated, which then creates the conduction through the bundle of His, the AV branches, and, finally, the Purkinje fibers. Once the impulse reaches the Purkinje fibers, the cardiac muscle that makes up the septum then contracts, which is rapidly followed by the contraction of the ventricles.

Electrical signals generated by the conduction of the heart's activity are recorded on the electrocardiograph machine by a series of waves, intervals, and segments, each of which pertains to a specific occurrence taking place during the conduction of the heart. These include the "P-wave," which represents the depolarization of the atrial myocardium; the "QRS-wave," sometimes called the "QRS complex," in which depolarization of the ventricular myocardium is taking place; the "P-R interval," representing the beginning of the excitation of the atrium to the beginning of the ventricular excitation; and the "S-T segment," which has no deflection from the baseline but in an abnormal state may be elevated or depressed. (See Figure 3–5.)

Electrical Conductivity

Electrical events occurring during the cardiac cycle can be considered as the cycle beginning with the "P-wave" in the electrocardiogram. At this point, the SA node has fired and the electrical current has begun to spread to the atrial myocardium. The atrium then depolarizes and contracts, which causes the P-wave in the electrocardiogram. During atrial systole, the atria contract, forcing blood from both atria into their respective ventricles. Next, the electrical current spreads to the AV node, bundle of His, and Purkinje fibers, during the interval from the end of the P-wave, until the "Q-wave" appears.

The entire process described above is called *atrial systole*. The "QRS" waves, which occur during this process, represent the depolarization of the ventricular myocardium, and it is during this period when the first heart sound is heard. This sound is the closing of the mitral and tricuspid valves. Also, during this period the ventricular pressure begins to increase, and when it reaches the systolic pressure the aortic valves open. After the "S-wave" and at the exact moment the aortic valves open, the heart cycle is in what we refer to as the *rapid ejection phase*. What occurs during this time is a rapid emptying of the ventricle, which in turn causes the arterial pressure to begin to rise to its highest level, and the

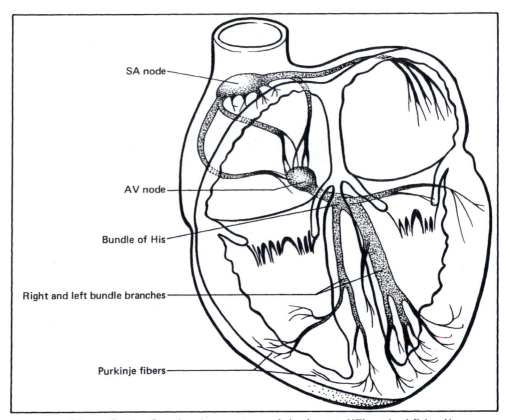

Figure 3–5 Conduction system of the heart. "Electrical firing" begins with the SA node, referred to as the "pacemaker," since all electrical impulses originate here before making their way through the rest of the heart.

ventricular myocardium, at the same time, to begin to make itself ready to repolarize, causing the "T-wave" to form the EKG.

At the end of the T-wave, the ventricle is beginning to relax and start ventricular diastole. At the exact time in which this is occurring, the arterial pressure in the aorta starts to exceed the pressure in the ventricle. The ventricle pressure then falls until such time as the atrial pressure exceeds the ventricular pressure. At that exact moment, the mitral and tricuspid valves open and the heart is in what we call the *rapid filling phase*. This phase is the time during which the ventricle fills up with blood. (See Figure 3–6.)

THE ELECTRICAL IMPULSE: UNDERSTANDING THE "PQRST COMPLEX"

The electrical activity in the heart that leads to the contraction of the heart muscle is displayed as a "PQRST pattern," or "complex" on the electrocardiographic paper. Each of these patterns, or complexes, represents the electrical activity occurring during the contraction phase

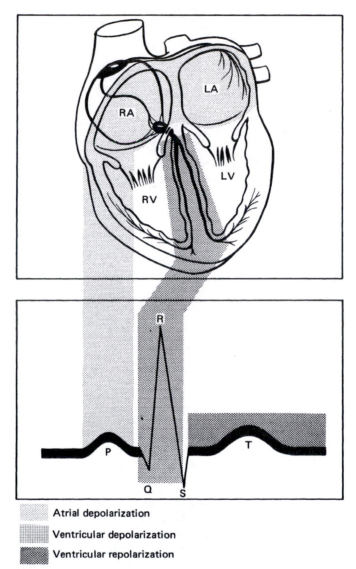

Atrial depolarization

Ventricular depolarization

Ventricular repolarization

Figure 3-6 Heart action in relation to EKG cycle.

of the heart muscle. Therefore, each PQRST phase represents one complete heartbeat.

A physician or trained health care professional can study the various parts of the complex and can determine any possible diseased or abnormal conditions present in the heart. Because of the importance of this pattern, it is extremely important that the technician make sure that this complex is centered on the paper and large enough so that all parts of it can be studied.

To make it easier for the technician to understand, let's take a look at the individual parts of the complex.

The P-wave, or the point at which depolarization begins to take place, indicates the spread of the impulse, generated by the SA node of the heart, over the atrium. It is therefore referred to as "depolarization of the atrium." The P-R interval is the period of time from the onset of the P-wave to the beginning of the "QRS-complex." This includes the time required for atrial depolarization and repolarization as well as the time necessary for the initial impulse from the SA node to arrive at the AV node.

The P-R segment represents the period of time from the end of the P-wave to the onset of the QRS-complex. Normally this is an isoelectric period on the EKG. The QRS-complex represents the electrical voltages during depolarization of the ventricles as the impulse begins to spread through the bundle of His, bundle branches, and Purkinje fibers. The S-T segment represents the interval between the end of the ventricular depolarization and the beginning of the ventricular repolarization. Physiologically, this is the interval between the ventricles contracting and their recovery. During the S-T interval, the ventricles also begin to recover from their contraction.

Finally, the Q-T interval represents the time interval from the beginning of ventricular depolarization to the completion of the ventricular repolarization. Physiologically, the Q-T interval represents the beginning of the ventricular contraction to the complete recovery of the ventricle. The U-wave, considered the "after-potential" of the T-wave, represents the repolarization of the ventricular Purkinje fibers. However, the precise significance of the U-wave is not completely known.

SUMMARY OF THE CARDIAC CYCLE

Now that we have discussed both the anatomy and the function of the cardiac cycle, let's try to summarize exactly what is happening during this most vital period. To begin with, the SA node, or the "pacemaker" of the heart, fires, causing both the atrium to contract and blood to be forced into the ventricles. The ventricular myocardium is then stimulated and contracts, causing the "lub," or first sound of the heartbeat, by the closing of the mitral and tricuspid valves, as a result of the increasing ventricular pressure.

Rapid ejection of blood from the ventricles into the arteries then takes place, causing the arterial pressure to rise to its maximum level, which in turn causes the ventricles to begin to relax. Arterial pressure is still high when the ventricular pressure begins to decrease. Immediately following this process, the "dub", or second sound emitted by the heartbeat, occurs as the pulmonary and aortic semilunar valves snap shut, thereby preventing blood from flowing back into the ventricles.

REVIEW QUESTIONS

Directions: For the questions below, give the answers you believe are most correct:

1. What is the primary function of all heart valves?

2. How many chambers are there in the heart?

3. What is the main function of the heart?

4. What is the largest artery in the body?

5. In what structure is the heart contained?

6. In the "lub-dub" sounds made by the heart, what does the "lub" represent? What does the "dub" represent?

7. Blood enters the _____ _____ from all parts of the body, and empties into the _____ _____ via the tricuspid valve.

8. The atrioventricular valves, which are located between the atrium and ventricles, include the _____ valve and the _____ _____ valve.

9. The _____ valves differ in their function from the atrioventricular, primarily because of their shape.

10. Briefly trace the flow of blood after it has been received by the right atrium:

11. Identify the three layers of the heart:

    (a) _____

    (b) _____

    (c) _____

12. Arteries carry _____ blood _____ from the heart.

13. Veins carry _____ blood _____ the heart.

14. The exchange between blood and oxygen takes place primarily within the

    _____ .

15. The two major ducts found in the lymphatic system include the _____

    _____ and the _____ .

16. _____ _____ pertains to the flow
    of blood taking place throughout the coronary arteries.

17. All cardiac muscle cells have an inherent, or characteristic, rate of con-

    traction called _____ .

18. During strenuous activity, the heart rate usually _____ .

19. A normal healthy adult heart beats aprpoximately _____ to _____
    beats per minute.

20. (a) Define the term *blood pressure:*

    (b) Define the term *systole:*

    (c) Define the term *diastole:*

Understanding the Role
of the EKG Technician

4

TERMINAL OBJECTIVE

To provide the student with an understanding of the role the EKG technician plays as a member of the health care delivery system.

COMPETENCY OBJECTIVES

Upon completion of this chapter, the student will be able to

1. Discuss the purpose of communication in the delivery of health care and identify the types of communication most often used in health care.
2. Discuss the role that observation plays in communication.
3. Describe the difference between verbal and nonverbal communication.
4. Discuss the EKG technician's role in possessing a professional and positive attitude.
5. Identify some of the more personal characteristics an EKG technician should possess.
6. Discuss the role safety plays in caring for the patient.
7. Discuss the principles of ethics and legal dimensions as they relate to the EKG technician.
8. Describe the difference between negligence and malpractice.

As a member of the medical community, the EKG technician is just as responsible for his or her own actions as are others who comprise the health care delivery system. Therefore, as with all health care provides, the role of the EKG technician involves working within an environment in which communication, professionalism, safety, and ethics are all of equal importance.

COMMUNICATION

Communication is defined as a two-way process in which information, facts, or feelings may be shared with others. Communication involves both a sender and a receiver, and it can be interpreted either in a verbal or nonverbal manner.

EKG technicians communicate with many people, including patients, co-workers, and with their supervisors within the health care environment. They are responsible for both transmitting and receiving information regarding the care and observation of the patient, as well as providing intercommunication among members of the hospital staff.

Observation

The process of observation takes on a particularly important role for the EKG technician, for much of what you will be involved in deals with the direct "hands-on" performance of tasks that measure the patient's most vital signs.

Observation means much more than just looking at a patient. It involves using all of your senses and noting anything that may appear unusual or out of the ordinary. It also utilizes the skills involved in communicating or reporting these findings to the person in charge of the patient or, in some cases, to your supervisor, or the physician, directly.

Your senses of vision and hearing are your two greatest assets in observing the patient. The more carefully and efficiently you make your observations, the more expertise you will develop in quickly identifying any situation that might be out of the ordinary.

The skills involved in observation do not come easily; they require both experience and practice. As you become more involved in these processes, you will begin to learn how to make "mental notes" automatically of what you see, feel, and access regarding the patient's condition. Eventually, you may even be able to sense a problem, or perhaps even change a negative situation into a positive one, before you ever discover its nature. Remember, to be of any value, observations must be communicated both effectively and efficiently.

Types of Communication

There are three types of communication you will be using in the health care setting. These include oral, or verbal communication, written communication, and nonverbal communication. (See Figure 4-1.)

Oral communication. Oral, or verbal communication, involves the utilization of both knowledge of what you are speaking about, as well as acceptable verbal skills necessary in communicating your message.

Two types of oral communication used most frequently in the hospital environment include answering the telephone and reporting information. While much of what the EKG technician does involves more physical performance of skills than it does verbal communication, there may be times when you are asked to use your expertise in oral communication. If, for example, you are asked to answer the telephone, you should always remember to identify the unit on which you are working as to give your name and your position. Providing callers with this information allows them to know immediately if they have reached the proper location, as well as knowing if you are the appropriate person to take the call.

The second type of oral communication used most frequently in the hospital is the use of oral reporting. This skill is employed most often to ensure that all members of the health care team fully understand the care that has been provided to the patient.

Whenever you are asked to give an oral report pertaining to a patient, you should always provide the person requesting the information with the name and location of the patient, the diagnosis or name of the condition or disorder for which the patient has been admitted to the hospital, the name of the physican caring for the patient, and any special instructions or information pertaining to the patient's condition that relates to the care or procedure that you have provided the patient.

Written Communication. There are two basic types of written communications in the hospital with which you may be involved. These include the patient's nursing care plan and the patient's medical chart.

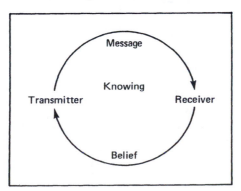

Figure 4-1   Circle of communication.

While nursing care plans are used primarily for the nursing care team, they also provide other members of the health care delivery team with a quick reference for checking pertinent information regarding the patient's diagnosis and care.

The medical chart is defined as a written record in which information regarding the patient is kept. Many members of the medical team, including the EKG technician, may be responsible for charting within this record. Therefore, you should understand that the chart, because it is considered a legal document, must be maintained in an accurate and efficient manner.

Every patient admitted to the hospital has a medical chart, which usually consists of several individual blanks that are later filled in with information about the patient. This will generally consist of a front sheet, with information regarding the patient's sex, marital status, admitting diagnosis, and employment; a history and physical form giving pertinent information regarding the patient's social and family history and the physical signs and symptoms he or she has been admitted to the hospital with; a daily progress report maintained by the patient's attending physician; a graphic chart used for recording the patient's vital signs; and nurses' notes, on which important information about the patient's daily care and treatment is recorded by the nursing staff. (See Figure 4–2.)

Other records, including blank pages for the patient's EKG tracing, laboratory work, and X-ray reports, may also be found within the medical record, depending upon the patient's condition and what tests may have been ordered for his or her care. In addition to being kept accurate and up-to-date, all records found in the patient's chart must be properly dated and must include the patient's name and hospital identification number, the name of the admitting physician, and the location or room number to which the patient has been assigned.

Nonverbal Communication. Nonverbal communication involves a process by which information or facts are communicated through the use of one's body gestures rather than through speech or writing. Commonly referred to as "body language," this type of communication can oftentimes tell more about a patient and how he or she is feeling than can verbal communication. A patient, for example, who is experiencing pain may be more apt to show signs of his or her discomfort by "holding" the affected area rather than by crying or talking about where the pain may be felt.

Nonverbal communication can be transmitted through a number of actions, including posture, hand or body movements, activity level, facial expressions, overall general appearance, and body position. And, just as the patient may communicate to you through his or her body movements, you should also remember that how you act and conduct yourself may also give meaning to the patient. Therefore, it is important that you be constantly aware of how you look and act to others. Simply making eye contact or gently touching the patient can take you one step closer to effectively communicating with the patient in a positive and caring way.

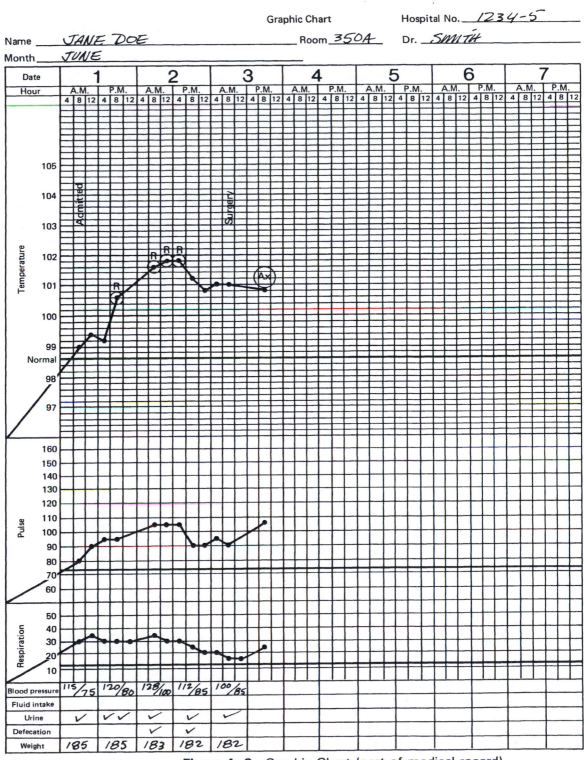

Figure 4-2 Graphic Chart (part of medical record).

PROFESSIONALISM AND ATTITUDE

Being an EKG technician requires that you possess both enthusiasm and a concerned and positive attitude for the profession of which you are a part. In addition, it requires that you not only be aware of the needs of others but that you carry yourself in a manner befitting a member of the health care delivery team. (See Figure 4–3.)

Professionalism involves those characteristics and personal traits that make up an individual who is committed to performing his or her job in an accurate and efficient manner. It includes having both a positive attitude and carrying oneself in a way in which others look to you for guidance and understanding of a "job well done."

The entire health care system is based upon meeting the needs of the patient. In order to accomplish this task, all members of the team must be keenly aware of not only what is expected of their individual position but also how they can best meet both the physical and psychosocial needs of the patient.

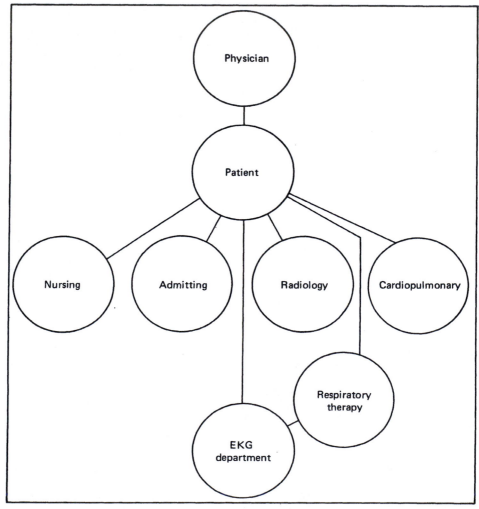

Figure 4–3 Health care delivery team.

Providing care and treatment to the hospital patient is based upon a delivery system and a chain of command, or line of authority. This requires that every member of the medical team carry out his or her respective tasks in order to provide all patients with the optimal care available.

The health care delivery team is made up of the nursing care team, who are individuals charged with carrying out the care and treatment of the patient; the auxiliary service departments, such as the EKG department, and the X-ray and laboratory departments, which perform specific tests necessary in the diagnosis of the patient; and the physician, the person who is ultimately responsible for seeing to it that the patient is both cared for and treated for an illness or disorder for which the patient has been admitted. In addition to carrying out their specific tasks, all members of the team are also responsible for seeing to it that they adhere to the strict guidelines and state and federal regulations set forth for the care and treatment of the patient.

Personal Characteristics

Just as important as seeing to the appropriate performance of one's own tasks is the way in which an individual carries oneself, including taking care of one's own health and hygiene. Good personal grooming, making sure your clothes or uniform is neat and clean, and maintaining a well-balanced, healthy diet are all essential to working within the health care profession. Taking a shower or bath daily, using deodorant, and avoiding the use of strong perfumes, as well as proper grooming of one's hair and fingernails, and eliminating the possibility of body odors such as tobacco smells, are all essential to working as a valued member of the health care team.

SAFETY AND CARE OF THE PATIENT

Just as important as the way in which you perform your skills and tasks, which are necessary to the patient's care and treatment, is the way in which these are carried out. Safety, above all, is the single most important task that all members of the health care team must observe.

You should remember that the patient's safety and comfort are everyone's concern. Always try to keep in mind that the needs and feelings of a patient involve maintaining a safe environment. This includes the patient's personal safety, such as making sure your equipment is in proper working order, as well as the safety of others, as in maintaining a clean and safe environment.

ETHICS AND THE EKG TECHNICIAN

The study of both ethics and the legal dimensions involved in working as an EKG technician within the health care system deals with having an understanding of those standards and principles inherent in the science and art of medicine. The code of ethics involved in health care deals with rules that act as guidelines for those individuals responsible for caring for the sick. These rules are both moral and legal and are grounded in the concept of the preservation of life.

Confidentiality

One of the most basic rules of ethics deals with what you—as a member of the health care team—see and hear while working in the health care facility. Much of the information you are concerned with is considered personal, and therefore it must be kept in strictest confidence. No matter how upset or distressed you might become, you must never allow yourself to discuss matters that concern patients, co-workers, or physicians. The medical code of ethics forbids any member of the health care team to discuss or repeat information concerned with the everyday workings of the hospital environment, particularly if it can be used for one's own personal gain. If you believe specific information is important to the welfare or concern of the patient, it should be reported through the appropriate channels as quickly as possible.

Patient Information

In some instances there may be times when a patient, or perhaps his or her visitors, question you as to the care or treatment being received. You must learn to evade graciously any questions not falling within your realm of responsibility. Questions and inquiries should be redirected to a physician or nurse who can properly and more concisely answer these questions. In addition, you should never discuss information concerning the death of a patient with family members, but rather refer any such inquiries to someone who is more informed on this subject. It is also a good idea not to get into the habit of discussing a patient's condition while in the patient's room, even if it appears that the patient is not responsive. Remember, the patient may be able to hear everything that is being said. (See Figures 4–4, 4–5, and 4–6.)

---

1. I authorized Dr. _____ to disclose complete information to _____ concerning medical findings and treatment of the undersigned from on or about _____ 19 _____ until date of the conclusion of such treatment.

2. Further, I authorized him/her to testify, without limitation, as to all of the medical findings and the treatment administered to the undersigned, in any legal action, suit, or proceedings to which I am, or may become, a party; and I waive, on behalf of myself and any persons who may have an interest in the matter, all provisions of law relating to the disclosure of confidential medical information.

Signed _____

Place _____

Date _____

Witness _____

Figure 4–4 Authorization for Disclosure of Information by Patient's Physician.

```
                                                            A.M.
Date _____  Time: _____  P.M.


    I authorize and request the _____ Hospital, and
the physician who attended me while I was a patient in said hospital
during the approximate period from _____ 19 ____
to _____ 19 _____ , to furnish to _____
all information concerning my case history and the treatment,
examination or hospitalization which I received, including copies of
hospital and medical records.

                              Signed _____


Witness _____
```

Figure 4–5 Authorization to Furnish Information.

```
I authorize Dr. _____ to disclose complete informa-
tion to _____ concerning the results of a physical
examination fo the undersigned made or to be made on _____
19_____ , and to testify, without limitation, as to all  findings of said
physical examination, in any legal action or  judicial  proceedings to
which I am, or may become, a party; and I waive on behalf of myself
and any persons who may have an interest in the matter, all provisions
of law relating to the disclosure of information acquired through said
examination.
```

Figure 4–6 Authorization for Disclosure of Information by
Examining Physician.

LEGAL DIMENSIONS

Negligence

The term *negligence,* when used in the medical sense, describes an individual failing to perform a task in a manner or in a way in which
another individual of the same training or background would perform
the task. Failing to make sure the EKG machine is in proper working
order before wheeling it into the patient's room to record the EKG tracing is one example in which an EKG technician would be guilty of
negligence.

Malpractice

Malpractice pertains to an individual performing a task for which he or
she has not been properly trained. One example would be an EKG technician recording the electrocardiogram on a patient prior to receiving
proper instruction on the techniques involved in its performance.

Reporting Inappropriate Acts

Because of the very nature of the work performed by members of the
health care team, individuals who are employed in hospitals and health
care facilities must possess the highest degree of honesty, dependabili-

ty, and integrity. This means that people working in medicine are expected to conduct themselves in an honest and professional manner. Therefore, anytime you are witness to such acts as the misuse of drugs, alcohol, or patient harm, you have both a moral and legal responsibility to report these acts.

Unfortunately, as a member of the health care team you will constantly be aware of the opportunities for poor practice, illegal activities, and the neglect of patients within the hospital environment. You should remember, however, that to be successful in your job, refraining from any activities that will make you suspect to illegal actions will not only increase your sense of honesty and integrity but also make you a valued member of the health care community. (See Figures 4–7 and 4–8.)

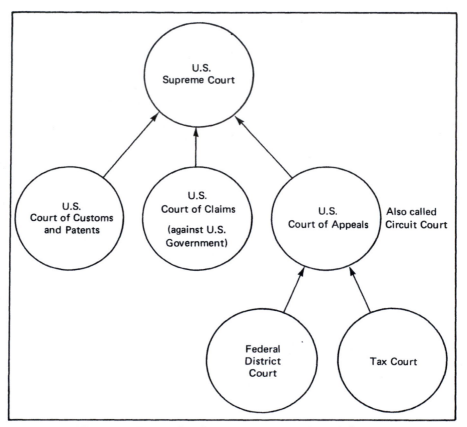

Figure 4–7   Judicial system in the United States.

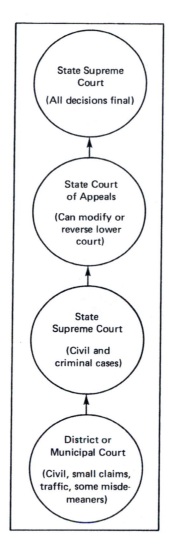

Figure 4–8 Typical state court system.

REVIEW QUESTIONS

Directions: For the questions below, give the answers you believe are most correct:

1. Define communication:

2. _____ involves using all of one's senses, and noting anything that may appear unusual or out of the ordinary.

3. Identify the three types of communication employed in the health care field:

    (a) _____

    (b) _____

    (c) _____

4. In order for communication to occur, there must be a _____ _____ and a _____ .

5. _____ and _____ are two examples of _____ communication in the hospital.

6. _____ communication involves a process by which information or facts are communicated through the use of one's body.

7. _____ involves those characteristics and personal traits which makeup an individual committed to performing his or her job in an accurate and efficient manner.

8. Identify at least five members of the health care team:

    (a) _____

    (b) _____

    (c) _____

    (d) _____

    (e) _____

9. The patient's _____ and _____ is everyone's responsibility and concern.

10. Define confidentiality:

11. Define ethics:

12. _____ deals with an individual failing to perform a task or job in the same manner in which another individual of the same training or background would perform the task.

13. _____ pertains to an individual performing a task for which he or she has not been properly trained.

14. _____ , _____ , and _____

_____ are three personal traits that all members of the health care team are expected to possess.

15. Identify at least two inappropriate acts performed in the hospital, which would constitute immediate reporting

(a) _____

(b) _____

Electrocardiographic
Equipment and Supplies

5

TERMINAL OBJECTIVE

To provide the student with an understanding of the different types of electrocardiographic equipment, machines, and supplies that are necessary to properly record an electrocardiogram.

COMPENTENCY OBJECTIVES

Upon completion of this chapter, the student will be able to

1. Correctly spell and define terminology related to EKG equipment and supplies.
2. Describe the purpose of the EKG machine and briefly explain how it operates.
3. Describe the purpose and techniques involved in properly "wiring" a patient for an electrocardiogram.
4. Discuss the general guidelines for proper placement of leads and electrodes (sensors) upon the patient's body.
5. Discuss the operation of the standard 12-lead EKG machine.
6. Explain the purpose of the individual switches and markers found on the standard 12-lead EKG machine.
7. Discuss the operation of the 3-channel computerized EKG machine.
8. Explain the purpose of the individual switches and markers found on the 3-channel computerized EKG machine.
9. Explain the purpose and use of EKG paper.
10. Explain the purpose and use of sensors and electrolyte.

THE EKG MACHINE

How the Machine Works

Before we discuss the actual skills involved in taking an electrocardiogram, it is extremely important that you first understand the parts of the EKG machine itself.

Although several different makes and models of EKG machines are currently in use, there are two basic classifications of machines that the majority of physicians and hospitals use to perform an electrocardiogram. These include the 12-lead EKG machine and the 3-channel EKG machine. For now, let's discuss the 12-lead machine.

The 12-lead EKG machine consists of five basic parts. These are the *electrodes,* which are made of small pieces of conductive metal used to pick up the electrical activity of the heart; the *leads,* which are wires responsible for carrying impulses from the electrodes that have been placed on the patient's skin and that are connected to the machine; the *amplifier,* whose purpose involves the magnification of the heart's electrical activity so that it can be recorded; the *galvanometer,* which converts the amplified electrical activity into motion; and the *stylus,* which records the motion onto the graph paper located in the machine. (See Figure 5–1.)

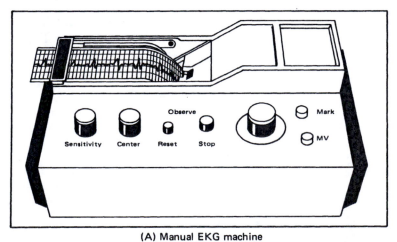

(A) Manual EKG machine

Figure 5–1 Two examples of elecrocardiographic machines currently in use.

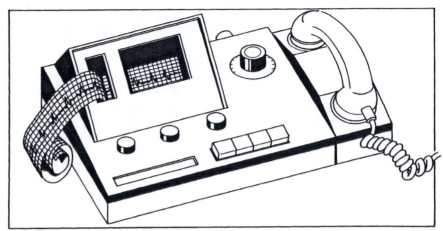

(B) EKG transmitted via phone lines

Figure 5–1 *(cont.)*

WIRING THE PATIENT

Whenver we discuss the use of an inanimate object such as an EKG machine being used as a tool in the treatment of a patient, it is extremely important that we also address the use of safety in terms of patient care. Because the EKG machine is an electrical instrument, precaution is doubly important, for improper use of the machine can have devastating effects on not just the patient's treatment but also on his or her complete state of health.

The most hazardous part of the EKG machine (which if not properly used could lead to a life-threatening situation) lies in the wires used to hook the patient up to the machine. While you will have ample opportunity to practice placing the electrodes on your patients during your training, the following information will help you to feel more at ease as you begin to learn how to "wire" the patient up correctly in order to perform the EKG tracing.

First of all, you should understand that the most critical aspect of the EKG procedure is the correct attachment of the electrodes and the leads, or the wiring of each from the patient to the machine. If either the electrodes or the leads are not placed correctly on the patient, the EKG graph will be both inaccurate and dangerous.

General Guidelines for Placement of Leads and Electrodes

Because safety is so very important in the correct placement of the leads and electrodes onto the patient during the taking of the EKG, the following general guidelines, or rules, have been provided for your understanding:

1. Prior to placing the leads and electrodes onto the patient, always wipe the patient's skin with a cleansing agent, especially if the skin is oily, scaly, or sweaty.

2. Always apply the electrode paste or conductive solution to the patient's arms and legs.

3. Remember that the arm electrodes are placed on the upper part of the arm. Use a *white* lead on the right arm and a *green* lead on the left arm.

4. Always remember to place the leg electrodes on the upper thighs. Use a *black* lead on the right leg and a *red* lead on the left leg. Remember:
   a. right arm (RA): WHITE
   b. left arm (LA): BLACK
   c. right leg (RL): GREEN
   d. left leg (LL): RED

5. Remember that there are six leads that must be placed upon the patient's chest, all of which have specific locations, and if the leads are placed incorrectly the EKG will be inaccurate. These leads include the following: *V1,* placed at the fourth intercostal (between the ribs) space, right sternal (breast bone) border; *V2,* placed at the fourth intercostal space, left sternal border; *V3,* placed equal distance between the V2 and V4 leads; *V4,* placed at the fifth intercostal space, left mid-clavicular (collar bone) line; *V5,* lateral (to the side) of the V4 lead, at the anterior (in front of) the axillary (arm pit) line; and *V6,* placed lateal to V5 at the mid-axillary line. Remember, correct placement is absolutely essential for accuracy and completeness in performing the EKG.

SWITCHES AND MARKERS

As we have already indicated, there are several different makes and models of EKG machines currently in use. However, all machines contain many of the same basic parts, including the switches and markers that make operation of the EKG possible. A good rule of thumb to remember is that whenever you are required to perform an electrocardiogram always check the manufacturer's instructions that accompany your machine prior to using it.

The Main Switch Control

The main switch control is used to turn the machine ON and OFF, and it should never be left in the ON mode when not in use.

The Pilot Light

The pilot light, usually seen as a red light on the machine, indicates that the machine is turned on. If you have turned the machine on and the light does not appear, there is a very good possibility that the machine may not be working properly. It should therefore be checked for correct operation prior to running the electrocardiogram.

Standard Control (ST'D)

The standard control (ST'D) allows the technician to standardize the machine. The machine thus cannot be operated without the use of a screwdriver. To standardize the machine, 1 millivolt electrical input should cause the stylus, or recording needle, or move 1 centimeter on the graph (10 small squares or 2 large squares on the paper). Turn the control clockwise in order to increase the size of the standard until it is at 10 small squares. Turning the control counterclockwise will decrease the size of the standard.

Stylus Head Control

The stylus head control is used to adjust the stylus temperature. The heat from the stylus melts the plastic coating on the EKG paper and forms the black line seen on the paper. At the same time, the coating lubricates the stylus. If the tracing is too light, the technician can use a screwdriver to turn the control clockwise, thereby increasing the heat and causing the tracing to become darker. If the line is too dark, turn the control back counterclockwise. The ideal proper setting is approximately one-quarter turn back from the full clockwise position.

Stylus Position Control

The stylus position control switch is used to move the recording up and down on the paper. In most cases, the control should be adjusted in order to center the EKG on the paper. (See Figure 5–2.)

Record Switch

The record switch has four separate functions, all of which are needed in order to control the amplifier and paper drive or the speed. These include the following:

1. Amp Off: This unit remains inactive and is used when changing the chest lead positions.
2. Amp On: Once the amplifier is activated, causing the stylus to move but the paper to remain stationary, this position

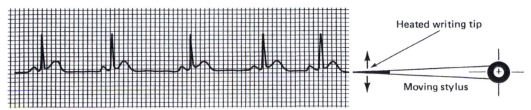

Figure 5–2   Heated wire tip and moving stylus.

is used for the chest leads. After the lead is in position, turn the machine to the Amp On and allow the stylus to stabilize or settle, and turn to "Run 25."

3. Run 25:   This is the position normally used when recording the EKG. It pertains to the paper moving at a rate of 25 millimeters (mm) per second.

4. Run 50:   The only time this position is normally used is when the complexes of the EKG are so close together that they are difficult for the physician or technician to examine. Its movement increases the speed of the paper to 50 mm per second and, therefore, stretches the EKG out onto the paper. Oftentimes it may be used to run an EKG tracing on a patient with an extremely fast heartbeat, or tachycardia. To make the physician aware of the increased speed, "Run 50" should be written on the paper with a pen or pencil.

Standardize Button (ST'D)

This button is used to put the standard mark onto the paper. It should be 10 small squares or 2 large squares high. This is extremely important to the physician, for the physician can determine the voltage produced by the heart only if the standard voltage is known.

Marker Button

The marker button is used to place a mark or code onto the paper in order to identify the lead being recorded. On some EKG machines, the marking may be done automatically; however, on others, the lead mark is recorded with this control at the start of each lead recording.

If the machine you are using does not automatically mark the leads, use the following codes to perform the marking manually:

1. . Lead 1   - . V1
2. .. Lead 2   - .. V2
3. ... Lead 3   - ... V3
4. - AVR   - V4
5. -- AVL   - V5
6. --- AVF   - V6

Lead Selector Switch

The lead selector switch allows the proper selection of the lead to be run.

Sensitivity Switch

The sensitivity switch controls the amplification and is usually set at the number "1." In the position "1," the standard is 10 small blocks or 2 large blocks high.

THE 3-CHANNEL COMPUTERIZED EKG MACHINE

As we have already discussed, there are two major classifications of EKG machines currently in use in most medical facilities and offices. They are the 12-lead manual EKG machine and the 3-channel computerized EKG machine. Although there are several different makes and models of the computerized system, the most frequently used is the Burdick E-310 microprocessor-based electrocardiograph machine.

This 3-channel computerized machine is a far cry from Einthoven's original massively built instrument. Unlike its predecessor, the E-310 machine was constructed with one goal in mind: to provide the physician with the most accurate, state-of-the-art analysis of the patient's heart, with the maximum amount of patient safety.

OPERATION AND CONTROLS

Like the 12-lead manual machine, the E-310 computerized machine also utilizes a number of controls that operate the machine.

Power Switch

The power switch is a two-position rocker switch and is responsible for turning the machine on and off. When the power switch is placed in the ON position, AC voltage is applied to the unit; placing the switch in the OFF position removes all power completely. Like the manual machine, the power switch should never be left in the ON position when not in operation.

Lead Select Switches

There are five switches that are provided for the technician, thus allowing the operator to select a particular lead group to be manually recorded. By momentarily pressing one of these switches, the technician may choose a specific lead group and illuminate the indicator in the switch. The selected lead group will then remain active until another *lead selector* switch or the STOP switch is pressed. The 000 switch causes a straight line to be recorded, which is of use in centering the stylus and checking calibrations.

Stop Switch

Pressing this switch will stop the paper drive, if it is moving, and reset the lead selection to 000. Any remaining switch selections will not be affected when the STOP switch is pressed.

Auto Run

When pressed, the AUTO RUN switch allows the paper to be queued in order to correct the starting point, thereby allowing a standard 12-lead EKG sequence to be recorded automatically. During this time, the speed, sensitivity, and filter position may not be changed. By pressing the STOP switch, the technician may then terminate the automatic sequence and thus allow the selection of another mode.

Man Run (Manual Run)

Pressing the MAN RUN switch on the E-310 machine activates the paper drive and thereby causes the unit to record the lead group selected by the LEAD SELECT switches.

1 mV Switch

This switch is used in conjunction with the 000 LEAD SELECT switch in order to test the gain and damping of the unit. When checking gain, the limb lead sensitivity will then determine the amplitude of the calibration pulse. If the 1 mV switch is continuously pressed, the calibration pulse will eventually decay in amplitude.

During an automatic sequence, the calibration pulse at the end of the EKG recording will be divided into two sections. The first section indicates the sensitivity selected for the limb leads, whereas the second section indicates the chest lead sensitivity.

Copy Opt

The COPY OPT switch is an option to the E-310 machine and is not required for operation. When this option is installed and the COPY OPT switch is pressed, the E-310 will then have the capacity to print a copy of the preceding automatic EKG or the last 10 seconds of the manual EKG information. This switch, however, cannot be functional when the option has not been installed onto the machine.

Speed 25/50

As with the 12-lead manual EKG machine, the paper drive can be adjusted to move at either 25 or 50 mm/second by pressing the appropriate switch. An indicator in the switch will light up, showing the selected speed.

Filter In/Out

This double-switch selection allows the technician to select the frequency response of the unit. When FILTER OUT is selected, the tracing will have maximum fidelity and the frequency response will meet or exceed the requirements of the American Heart Association. If a recording shows signs of interference from muscle voltage, AC, or similar artifacts, the FILTER IN switch should be pressed. This will then filter out a majority of the unwanted artifacts from the tracing. An indicator will light in the appropriate switch, thereby showing the selected mode.

Chest × ½ Switch

When this switch is pressed, the chest sensitivity or amplitude will be reduced by one-half. This means that an input of 10 mm will result in a trace amplitude of 5 mm. By pressing this switch a second time, the sensitivity will return to × 1. The chest lead sensitivity is automatically set to × 1 when the unit is turned to ON. An indicator in the switch will light when the × ½ has been selected.

Limb × ½ , × 1, × 2 Switch

Limb lead sensitivity (leads 1, 2, 3, AVF, AVL, and AVR) can be selected by pressing the desired switch. A sensitivity of × 1 will automatically be selected when the unit is turned to the ON position. An indicator will light in the appropriate switch, showing the selected sensitivity.

Position

The three controls that make up the POSITION switch are responsible for adjusting the position of the recording styluses in their respective channels. By rotating the control upwards, the stylus will move up; rotating it downwards will move the stylus down.

Stylus Heat

This control is provided with a screwdriver slot in order to prevent inadvertent adjustment. It is preset at the factory in order to produce a solid clean line on the recording paper, when the paper speed is 25 mm/ second. The proper setting is approximately one-third back from the full counterclockwise position. Rotating the control clockwise increases the stylus heat; rotating it in the opposite direction will cause the stylus heat to decrease. Once this adjustment is properly set, it seldom requires subsequent adjustment.

Power Connection Cable

As with the 12-lead manual EKG machine, the E-310 machine is also supplied with a power cable. Connecting the cable from the power jack on the rear panel to a properly grounded wall outlet allows the unit to become automatically grounded.

Patient Cable

Both the E-310 machine and the 12-lead manual EKG machine utilize a PATIENT CABLE cord, which is the mainline connection between the patient and the machine. Care must be used with both units to ensure the proper safety and function of this cord, for any malfunction could cause either inaccuracy of the recording or prove hazardous to the patient's safety.

EKG Paper

Although the 3-channel computerized EKG machine may use a different size and type of paper from that used by the standard 12-lead machine, all EKG paper is treated in such a way as to react to the stylus heat so that a tracing can be produced upon the paper.

Electrocardiographic paper is designed to be divided into two sets of squares. Its sole purpose is to provide for total accuracy and measurement of the electrical waves, intervals, and segments as they relate to the recording of the patient's heartbeat. Each square of the paper is made up of 25 smaller squares, with each one measuring 1 millimeter (mm) high and 1 millimeter wide. When measured horizontally, each square represents the time in which each beat of the heart is recorded—that is, 0.04 seconds per square. When the square is measured vertically, each represents the amount of voltage being fired off by the heart—that is, 0.1 millivolts (mV) per square.

All electrocardiographic paper consists of a black base overlying a white plastic coating. It is made that way so that when the heated stylus moves over it a reaction occurs, causing the paper to melt, or break down the plastic coating, leaving only the recording of the tracing. In addition to the paper being coated with plastic, it is both heat and pressure sensitive, thereby allowing the stylus of the EKG machine to produce a clear and sharp image of the tracing. (See Figure 5–3.)

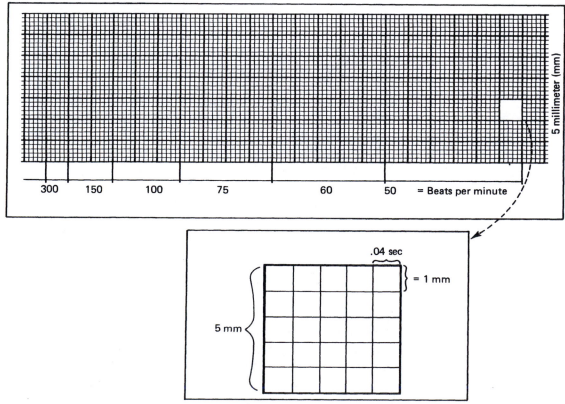

Figure 5–3 EKG paper.

SENSORS AND ELECTROLYTE

As previously indicated, sensors are used to attach the patient to the lead, which in turn connects the patient to the EKG machine. In essence, the main purpose of a sensor is to act as a conductor so that the machine can record the electrical impulses made by the heart and eventually record them onto the paper of the EKG machine.

The most frequently used sensors are called *Welsh self-retaining* sensors, and they are included as part of the standard accessories supplied with the electrocardiograph machine. While this type is most commonly used with the E-310 machine, a good rule of thumb is to never mix sensors with those of another manufacturer; the metal of which they are made may be dissimilar, and considerable baseline drifting or blocking, may result. (See Figure 5–4.)

An *electrolyte* is used to assist the machine in creating conductivity from the sensor, which has been attached to the patient and to the machine, so that electrical currents or impulses produced by the heart can be traced. Some machines, like the E-310, may use a liquid electrolyte; the liquid provides excellent conductivity between the patient's skin and the sensors. Other EKG machines, such as the Burdick EK/5A standard 12-lead, may use either the liquid electrolyte or electrolyte pads, which are gently attached to the inside of the sensor and then removed after the tracing is completed.

No matter what type of electrolyte is used, it is important to make sure that you wipe the sensors clean after each application. Preferably, the sensors should be washed after use and then scoured frequently with a kitchen cleanser. Excessive corrosion or an accumulation of electrolyte

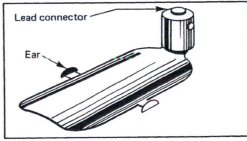

(A) Flat plate sensor

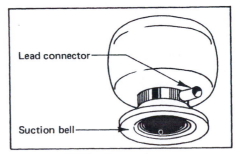

(B) Suction cup sensor

Figure 5–4 Limb sensors.

may cause the baseline to drift and thereby impair the quality of the EKG tracing.

Sensor Application

When using a liquid electrolyte, the following guidelines will assist the technician in the proper application of the sensors:

1. Expose the arms, legs, and chest of the patient.
2. Connect the patient leads to the self-retaining sensors; that is, 10 sensors for a standard 12-lead EKG.
3. Squeeze a small amount of electrolyte onto the sensor site and use the sensor to spread it evenly over the sensor contact area. Always make sure you apply the same amount of electrolyte to each sensor site. Depress the rubber bulb slightly when applying the sensor so as to leave only a small dimple when the bulb is released.
4. For the arm sensors, position the sensor on a smooth, fleshy area of the upper arm. Position so that the sensor will not press against the body or table when the patient is relaxed. By placing the sensor on the upper arm, muscle tremor artifacts will be minimized. The sensor site may be cleansed with an alcohol swab if oily skin conditions exist.
5. Attach the leg sensors on a fleshy part of the lower leg, but not over the tibia.
6. Attach the six chest sensors in the positions indicated in the Lead Arrangement and Coding Chart.
7. Be sure the leads conform to the body's contours, with no strain placed on the sensors. Avoid looping any excess length of lead wire.
8. Plug the patient cable into the patient jack unit until it is secure.

UNDERSTANDING DIFFERENT TYPES OF EKG RECORDING EQUIPMENT

Although the majority of electrocardiographic recordings the EKG technician may come in contact with deal mostly with the manual or standardized 12-lead machines, there are many variations of equipment the physician may choose to use to meet the individual needs of the patient.

THE MINI-HOLTER TRANSTELEPHONIC SYSTEM

The Mini-Holter Transtelephonic System, manufactured by the Holter Data Services Company, was developed to provide physicians with a means by which they could monitor a patient's EKG over a 24-hour period. The main advantage of using this type of device over a standard 12-lead EKG machine is that it reports continuous analysis, giving the physician important diagnostic data in environments that were previously not available. Thus, the system allows constant ambulatory monitoring of the patient for as many days as the physician determines is necessary. (See Figure 5–5.)

Parts of the System

The Mini-Holter System consists of two main parts: (1) the Holter EKG Recorder, which weighs approximately 5 ounces and is about one-fourth the size of a standard Holter Monitor, and (2) the Holter Data Bank Report Generator, which fits into the memory bank of any IBM XT-compatible computer system. The primary function of these two parts is to analyze each EKG continuously, selecting pertinent two-lead recordings for storage into its solid-state memory. While the recording period can be fixed anywhere from 24 hours to several weeks, depending upon the physician's discretion, programming can also be established within the device to record S-T segment changes, ventricular ectopic beats, couplets, ventricular tachycardia, and pauses. If no abnormalities are detected, it will also record normal EKG strips. (See Figure 5–6.)

General Supplies for the Mini-Holter System

In addition to the IBM XT-compatible computer system, certain general supplies are necessary in order to use the Mini-Holter System. These include standard 9-volt alkaline batteries and a set of five individual electrodes, which are compatible for use with the Mini-Holter.

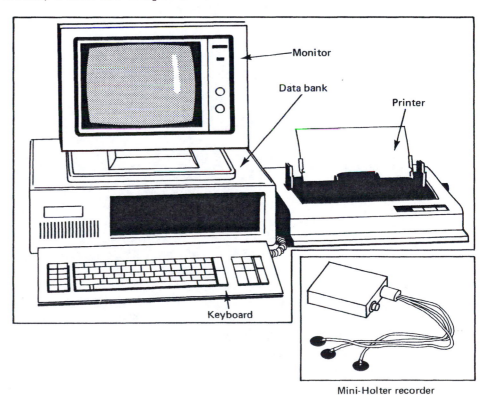

Figure 5–5 Mini-Holter data bank system.

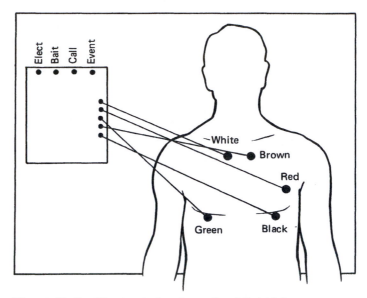

Figure 5–6   Electrode hook-up for Mini-Holter system.

Accessories Needed For the Mini-Holter System

Accessories.   Accessories for the Mini-Holter System include an electrode lead wire set, electrodes (five per procedure), alcohol preps, scrubs, and a razor.

Paper.   A Dot-Matrix printer must be used in order to record EKG strips with the Mini-Holter. The paper that the printer uses must be $9\frac{1}{2}$-by-11-inch and should be a 20-pound-bond type.

PREPARING THE MINI-HOLTER SYSTEM

As an EKG technician it is most important that you understand that the quality of the EKG data transmission is directly dependent upon how well the electrodes are applied to the patient. Because this system works, for all intents and purposes, on its own, and because the technician will not be able to be at the patient's side for every hookup, it is imperative that the patient fully understands the complete procedure for hooking up this system before affixing the electrodes of the Mini-Holter to their positioning sites on the patient.

As with the standard 12-lead EKG system, both the location and the manner in which the electrodes are set up on the Mini-Holter System are extremely important. Figure 5–6 indicates the positioning site of the five electrodes. Once the EKG technician has determined where the electrodes are placed, he or she should follow the steps outlined below:

1. Thoroughly clean the patient's skin where the electrodes are to be placed.
2. Shave any hair from the electrode site.

3. Scrub the electrode site with a prep pad.
4. Remove the backing on the electrode and place it on the chest. Press the center of the electrode and work out toward the edge.
5. The electrode lead wire set is color-coded. The colors (white, red, green, brown, and black) correspond to the colors on the Mini-Holter jacks.
6. Place the lead wire (male end) into the female pin by color-matching it to the Holter Recorder.
7. Snap the other end of the lead set to each corresponding color electrode on the chest.
8. Install a new 9-volt battery in the Holter Recorder. Five "beeps" will indicate that the power is on.
9. If the electrode buzzer beeps 20 times and there is no electrode LED flash, an electrode disconnect has occurred. Check and connect a lead wire, and make certain that no electrode has been removed from the patient.

Preparing the Patient

As with any procedure requiring the patient's understanding, always remember to explain what the purpose of this procedure is. Discuss and review the different parts of the system with the patient, and always ask the patient if he or she has any questions. A little bit of explanation goes a long way in lessening anxieties and frustrations the patient may be experiencing.

OPERATING THE MINI-HOLTER SYSTEM

Once you have explained the procedure to the patient you are ready to begin operation of the EKG.

The Mini-Holter is a system that transmits the patient's EKG data via the telephone, from the Holter Recorder to the Holter Data Bank. An S-T level may be changed per the physician's preference, and is normally preset at 80 mm/second (1.5 mm). To set the S-T level, the technician simply removes the four screws located at the back of the recorder and unhooks the top lid from it. Switches can then be moved to make the change of setting. Once the indicator has been changed, the lid is replaced and all four screws are tightened.

Transmitting the Data

Because this system works through the telephone, transmitting the EKG recording is extremely important. To transmit the recording do the following:

1. Dial the transmitter telephone number, which is located in the patient's chart.

2. After a few rings, a "squeal" tone can be heard. If this tone is not heard, phone back in about 15 minutes.

3. Place the phone mouthpiece on the Holter and directly over the company's printed name (Holter Data Services). Hold the recorder firmly to the mouthpiece.

4. Slide the transmitter switch to ON.

5. After several minutes a continuous loud tone will be heard, indicating that the Holter transmission is complete.

6. Slide the transmit switch to the OFF position.

7. Wait for the five "beep" tones.

8. Remove the telephone from the face of the recorder and hang up the telephone.

OTHER EKG MACHINES

Now that we have discussed the three primary modes of recording an electrocardiogram—that is, through the use of the standardized 12-lead EKG machine, the 3-channel E-310 computerized EKG machine, and the portable Mini-Holter ambulatory system—let's go back to what we first stated at the beginning of this chapter, namely that there are several different makes and models of EKG machines currently on the market that are being used in hospitals and in physicians' offices.

To begin this discussion it is important first to note that the two largest manufacturers of EKG machines are the Burdick Company and the Birtcher Corporation. Because the majority of machines that the EKG technician will be using are those primarily made by the Burdick Company, our discussion will focus first on those Burdick systems most commonly in use.

Presently, Burdick manufactures seven different types of machines used to measure and record electrocardiograms. These include the EK10, the Elite, the E-310, the ExTol/320, the E500 TW, the E600, and the ExTOL 300.

The EK10

The EK10 is a single-channel EKG machine with an optional EKG tracing that is built in. This machine is the most common standardized manual 12-lead recorder currently in use in most medical offices; it is capable of giving a full, mountable EKG in 37.5 seconds. In addition to the rapid time in which it delivers the recording, this particular model houses its own mount, which can be completed in either a single-channel or 3-channel format.

The Elite

Burdick's Elite Model EKG machine produces single-channel EKGs with interpretations that are considered highly accurate. In addition to its ability to produce the interpretation of the EKG strip, this machine is also capable of mounting the rhythm strip on its own cards.

The E-310

This microprocessor-based recorder is perhaps the single most popularly used computerized system responsible for simplifying 3-channel EKG technology. Designed to produce diagnostically accurate records with maximum definition and fidelity, this system is considered to be one of the leaders in terms of cost-effectiveness, due in large part to its functional simplicity and high productivity.

In terms of recording the actual EKG strips, the E-310 is capable of producing a 3-channel resting EKG. By doing so, it is able to give the physician a more accurate look at the patient's heart. What makes the E-310 even more productive is its ability to function in both an automatic and a manual mode.

The ExTOL/320

While the ExTOL/320 closely resembles both the size and the shape of the E-310, its capability is much greater, because it is constructed to meet the demands for the stress-testing procedures.

The ExTOL/320 is Burdick's latest 3-channel EKG machine, specifically designed for simplicity of operation, high volume, and efficient performance in tests of exercise tolerance. It is considered to be both operator- and patient-friendly, and it also has the capability to interface with an IBM personal computer for data collection, measurement, and report generation.

The E500 TW

The E500 TW is considered to be Burdick's "top of the line" machine for nonstress, 3-channel, interpretative EKG monitoring. Adding to its highly accurate yet simple design, the E500 TW has a recorder that can be removed for easier portability. The recorder can also store and retrieve 20 to 40 EKGs, acquire patient data, and give back interpretations and the measurements on which the recordings are based.

Considered to be a high-tech, state-of-the-art system, the E500 TW is capable of many functions. It can deliver pertinent patient and demographic information, provide interpretations of EKG measurements, and contains a directory that lists all EKGs that have been saved; a medication/blood pressure directory that lists two medications and diastolic blood pressure values that can be appended to each patient's EKG record; a "real time" monitoring system, which uses an LCD to monitor any lead in REAL TIME, and Median Complex Waveforms, which show EKG data from 12 classical leads, in order to derive a Median QRS Complex Waveform, in 10 seconds' time.

Perhaps the greatest attribute of the E500 TW is its ability to produce single-source documentation of the patient's EKG data. It does so by producing a Physician's Summary, which presents all data on a ready-to-file, $8\frac{1}{2}$-by-11-inch report that includes the patient's name and identification number, age, height, weight, sex, race, and blood pressure. The form also lists up to two medications that the patient may be taking, the time and date the EKG is being recorded, the ventricular rate, and the P-R interval, QRS duration, P-R-T axis measurement, and the QT and QT corrected.

The E600

Another EKG machine that Burdick manufactures is the E600, which is very similar to the E500 TW except that it is designed for stress-testing, and the recorder is not removable.

The ExTOL 300

The ExTOL 300 utilizes fully automatic protocol sequencing with physician-designated print intervals for 12-lead and 10-second rhythm strip printouts. Considered the "top of the line" for stress-testing, the ExTOL 300 includes the E320 3-channel EKG recorder, a heavy-duty treadmill, and a monitor/treadmill controller. Its operation is considered to be patient-focused, with minimal interaction by the EKG technician. It has an 18-stage, customized exercise capability, or one of six pre-programmed stress protocols. In addition to the highly accurate performance of this machine, the ExTOL 300 is capable of providing dual EKG diagnostics in either a resting or stress mode.

Although the Burdick Company, with its various types of EKG machines, is considered to be the leader in the EKG monitoring industry, the Birtcher Corporation has also produced a machine that is similar to Burdick's EK10.

Considered to be an excellent unit for the training of EKG technician students (because of its simple design), the Cardiotracer is a single-channel, noninterpretative unit with basic abilities. However, the single most negative attribute of this machine deals with its cable. While it is smaller in diameter than Burdick's EK10, it also adds to its "tangle tendency," making it a more time-consuming instrument for use by more advanced technicians.

REVIEW QUESTIONS

Directions: For the questions below, give the answers you believe would be most
correct:

1. Identify the two basic classifications of EKG machines currently in use by
the majority of physicians and hospitals:

    (a) _____

    (b) _____

2. Identify the five basic parts of the EKG machine:

    (a) _____

    (b) _____

    (c) _____

    (d) _____

    (e) _____

3. What part of the EKG machine is considered to be the most hazardous if
not properly used?

4. What is the most critical aspect of the EKG procedure?

5. Match the correct electrodes to the appropriate leads:

    (a) RA _____   1. Red

    (b) LA _____   2. Black

    (c) RL _____   3. Green

    (d) LL _____   4. White

6. Identify the correct placement of each of the chest leads:

    (a) V1 _____

    (b) V2 _____

    (c) V3 _____

    (d) V4 _____

    (e) V5 _____

    (f) V6 _____

7. Identify the function of each of the following controls:

    (a) Pilot light: _____

    (b) Standard control: _____

    (c) Stylus head control: _____

    (d) Stylus position control: _____

8. The _____ switch controls the amplification and is usually set at the number "1."

9. On the E-310 EKG machine, what does the "speed 25/50" switch represent?

10. The _____ _____ is the main-line connection between the patient and the EKG machine.

11. Each square of EKG paper is made up of _____ smaller squares, measuring one _____ high and one _____ _____ wide.

12. EKG paper is both _____ and _____ sensitive.

13. _____ is used to assist in creating the conductivity from the sensor, attached to the patient, to the EKG machine.

14. Excessive corrosion accumulated by the _____ may cause the baseline to _____ , thereby impairing the quality of the EKG tracing.

Patient Preparation: Meeting the Physical and Psychosocial Needs of the Cardiac Patient

6

TERMINAL OBJECTIVE

To provide the student with an understanding of the purpose and skills involved in meeting both the physical and psychosocial needs of the cardiac patient.

COMPETENCY OBJECTIVES

Upon completion of this chapter, the student will be able to

1. Identify the most basic of all human needs.
2. Discuss how the EKG technician may effectively deal with a frightened patient.
3. Discuss how the EKG technician may effectively deal with and meet the patient's physical needs.
4. Discuss the cardiac patient's Bill of Rights, and briefly identify each of those rights that are inherent in the care of all hospital patients.

All of us require necessities in life in order to help us get along and interact with others. These needs are both physical, such as requiring heat when the weather is cold, and emotional, as in needing love and understanding. For cardiac patients, who may be experiencing feelings of despair, believing their life may be over, meeting the patient's everyday physical needs and helping provide them with emotional and psychological support can make the difference between total recovery from a cardiac condition and death.

Human beings grow—that is, change physically and develop psychologically—throughout their entire lives. In affect, all of us go through life on a continuum that begins at birth and ends with death. Not all people, however, progress at the same rate in their growth and development, and it is for this reason that the provision of both physical and emotional well-being is so vitally important to the hospitalized cardiac patient.

UNDERSTANDING HUMAN NEEDS

Psychological or developmental skills and physical growth vary throughout one's life; however, it is our basic human needs—that is, the need to communicate, to have one's emotional and spiritual well-being assured, and to have specific physical needs, such as food, shelter, clothing, etc., fulfilled—that are paramount to our very existence.

Everyone wants to be understood by others. We all want to be able to communicate what we feel. We meet this need to communicate both verbally and through the use of nonverbal signals, such as crying or changing our facial expressions. In addition to communicating our feelings, human beings have a great need to experience emotional well-being. In doing so, we both enhance and protect our self-esteem. In health care, how patients respond to threats on their self-esteem depends upon how they interpret their own feelings of helplessness before, during, and after their illness.

DEALING WITH THE FRIGHTENED PATIENT

In order to deal with the frightened or fearful patient, it is important to first recognize that he or she is a person with both likes and dislikes. Crying and fearfulness may be a way in which the patient "acts out" a feeling of pain or despair. For the person suffering from a cardiac dysfunction, the constant threat of death and the pain and discomfort felt by the patient may force the patient to cry for what appears to be no reason at all. Being able to understand and recognize the patient's fears and anxieties will help you to more effectively communicate your desire to assist the patient during bouts with sadness and fright.

DEALING WITH THE PATIENT'S PHYSICAL NEEDS

In addition to the basic needs we all require to survive—that is, food, shelter, sleep, etc.—the cardiac patient may require special physical care in order to survive. Part of the responsibility of being a member of the health care team is to be aware of these needs, particularly as they relate to special procedures the patient may be undergoing as part of his or her care and treatment. Whether it is providing privacy during the recording of the EKG tracing or support to a family outside a patient's room, the EKG technician's role is not only to perform the basic tasks involved in one's job but, just as important, also to assist the rest of the team members in helping to meet the very special physical needs of the cardiac patient.

THE CARDIAC PATIENT'S RIGHTS

All patients who are hospitalized, whether they are suffering from a cardiac dysfunction or are admitted long enough to deliver a baby, are entitled to have their basic rights observed. This means that they have the right to know and understand that all orders the physician writes will be followed accurately and that procedures will be carried out properly and according to the way in which they should be. It also means that the patient has a right to be properly identified, according to his or her name, and to be provided with a sense of security every time you check the patient's nameband prior to carrying out a procedure.

Because the rights of patients being admitted to the hospital are so very important, the American Hospital Association on February 6, 1973, issued what is known as the "Patient's Bill of Rights." This document states the following:*

1. The patient has the right to considerate and respectful care.
2. The patient has the right to obtain from his† physician complete current information concerning his diagnosis, treatment, and prognosis in terms the patient can be reasonably expected to understand. When it is not medically advisable to give such information to the patient, the information should be made available to an appropriate person in his behalf. He has the right to know, by name, the physician responsible for coordinating his care.
3. The patient has the right to receive from his physician information necessary to give informed consent prior to the start of any procedure and/or

*Reprinted with permission of the American Hospital Association, © 1972.
†Single-sex pronouns reflect the wording in the American Hospital Association document.

treatment. Except in emergencies, such information for informed consent should include but not necessarily be limited to the specific procedure and/or treatment, the medically significant risks involved, and the probable duration of incapacitation. Where medically significant alternatives for care or treatment exist, or when the patient requests information concerning medical alternatives, the patient has the right to such information. The patient also has the right to know the name of the person responsible for the procedures and/or treatment.

4. The patient has the right to refuse treatment to the extent permitted by law and to be informed of the medical consequences of his action.

5. The patient has the right to every consideration of his privacy concerning his own medical care program. Case discussion, consultation, examination, and treatment are confidential and should be conducted discreetly. Those not directly involved in his care must have the permission of the patient to be present.

6. The patient has the right to expect that all communications and records pertaining to his care should be treated as confidential.

7. The patient has the right to expect that within its capacity a hospital must make reasonable response to the request of a patient for services. The hospital must provide evaluation, service, and/or referral as indicated by the urgency of the case. When medically permissible, a patient may be transferred to another facility only after he has received complete information and explanation concerning the needs for and alternatives to such a transfer. The institution to which the patient is to be transferred must first have accepted the patient for transfer.

8. The patient has the right to obtain information as to any relationship of his hospital to other health care and educational institutions insofar as his care is concerned. The patient has the right to obtain information as to the existence of any professional relationships among individuals, by name, who are treating him.

9. The patient has the right to be advised if the hospital proposes to engage in or perform human experimentation affecting his care or treatment. The patient has the right to refuse to participate in such research projects.

10. The patient has the right to expect reasonable continuity of care. He has the right to know in advance what appointment times and physicians are available and where. The patient has the right to expect that the hospital will provide a mechanism whereby he is informed by his physician or a delegate of the physician of the patient's continuing health care requirements following discharge.

11. The patient has the right to examine and receive an explanation of his bill regardless of the source of payment.

12. The patient has a right to know what hospital rules and regulations apply to his conduct as a patient.

The American Hospital Association further states that

No catalogue of rights can guarantee for the patient the kind of treatment he has a right to expect. A hospital has many functions to perform, including the prevention and treatment of disease, the education of both health professionals and patients, and the conduct of clinical research. All these activities must be conducted with an overriding concern for the patient, and, above all, the recognition of his dignity as a human being. Success in achieving this recognition assures success in the defense of the rights of the patient.

REVIEW QUESTIONS

Directions: For the questions below, give the answers you believe are most correct:

1. List at least three physical necessities of life:

   (a) _____

   (b) _____

   (c) _____

2. List at least two psychological or emotional necessities of life:

   (a) _____

   (b) _____

3. What is the most basic need of all human beings?

4. In order to deal with a frightened or fearful patient, it is important to first

   be able to _____ his _____ and

   _____ .

5. What are two fears the cardiac patient is most frightened of?

   (a) _____

   (b) _____

6. Caring for the cardiac patient's _____ needs are just as important as caring for his physical and emotional needs.

7. All hospitalized patients are entitled to their _____ rights.

8. It is important to ensure the patient's _____ whenever recording an EKG tracing.

9. On what date did the American Hospital Association institute the "Patient's Bill of Rights"?

10. How many "rights" are contained within the "Patient's Bill of Rights"?

Performing
Electrocardiography

7

TERMINAL OBJECTIVE

To provide the student with a basic understanding of the concepts, skills, and techniques involved in properly recording and mounting the standard 12-lead electrocardiogram and the 3-channel computerized electrocardiogram.

COMPETENCY OBJECTIVES

Upon completion of this chapter, the student will be able to

1. Correctly spell and define terminology related to properly recording and mounting a standard 12-lead electrocardiogram and a 3-channel computerized electrocardiogram.
2. Explain the purpose and function of the standard 12-lead electrocardiogram.
3. Describe the proper procedure involved in correctly recording and mounting the standard 12-lead electrocardiogram.
4. Explain the purpose and function of the 3-channel computerized electrocardiogram.
5. Describe the proper procedure involved in correctly recording and mounting the 3-channel computerized electrocardiogram.
6. Describe the safety precautions necessary whenever the EKG technician is required to record and mount either a standard 12-lead electrocardiogram or a 3-channel computerized electrocardiogram.

UNDERSTANDING THE ELECTROCARDIOGRAM

As we have previously discussed, an electrocardiogram, or EKG, is defined as a picture or tracing of the electrical current, or impulses, occurring in the human heart. During the electrocardiographic procedure, an electrode—that is, a metal alloy conductor placed upon the patient's skin—is responsible for both receiving and conducting the electrical impulses being "fired off" by the heart's conduction system. By using these special electrodes, the electrical activity is then recorded from different angles, which are called *leads*. The different leads, or angles, give the physician a more complete picture of the heart. By noting an electrical disturbance in any of the leads, the doctor can then determine which parts of the heart may be diseased or malfunctioning.

A complete EKG normally consists of 12 leads, with the electrodes being placed at specific locations on the body in order to pick up the voltage present.

An electrocardiogram, or EKG, is considered a relatively simple procedure, and it is used most frequently to help the physician to detect any abnormalities involving the heart's action. In fact, the term *electrocardiogram* is used to define any electrical record of the heart's activity.

The EKG is used to record the electrical impulses of the heart as the blood is pumped through the body. Tracings of electrical impulses appear as "waves" on a graph paper, creating a wave pattern reflecting the continuous phases of contractions and relaxations of the heart's four chambers.

Why the EKG is Important

The use of the electrocardiogram is a very effective way of detecting heart disease and abnormalities, and it is primarily used as a diagnostic tool in determining the status of the patient's heart. It may also be used as an invasive tool, in assisting the physician to rule out any other problems associated with the heart.

Heart and cardiovascular diseases affect more than 40 million Americans every year, and if diagnosed early, many heart problems can be successfully treated before they have had the chance to become acute and life-threatening.

Why an EKG May Be Ordered by the Physician

A physician is compelled to order an electrocardiogram whenever he or she believes the patient's symptoms might indicate an impending heart problem. When such symptoms occur, an EKG will help the physician to diagnose the cause of the problem and will then assist in the determination of the right course of treatment.

In addition to the EKG being used as a diagnostic tool in determining treatment of a cardiac or cardiovascular disease, the procedure may also be performed as a means of treatment in other instances. Patients who have already suffered a heart attack, for example, must have an EKG taken after the onset in order to determine the exact cause of the attack. In this case, the procedure helps the physician to assess just how much damage occurred to the heart as a result of the attack.

Patients who have a history of previous heart problems or heart attacks are also given an EKG routinely as a means of observing their present state of health. In this case, the EKG helps the physician to monitor the patient's condition and assists in detecting any improvement or deterioration in the patient's condition.

Many cardiac patients are required to take certain medications on a routine basis in order to help their heart to continue to beat strongly and efficiently. When a prescribed medication is ordered by the physician, he or she normally orders that an EKG be done on the patient so as to evaluate the effects of the medication and to check for any side effects.

Finally, an electrocardiogram may also be ordered as part of a routine checkup, either in the physician's office or when the patient is admitted to the hospital for observation, treatment, or surgery. In this case, the procedure is ordered so that the patient's medical history is kept current, so as to reassure the patient this his or her heat is in good condition, and to help the physician in the detection of any early signs or symptoms of impending heart disease.

PERFORMING THE ELECTROCARDIOGRAM

Preliminary Steps for Performing the 12-Lead EKG

Now that we have discussed both the equipment used in performing the manual 12-lead EKG, as well as the basic skills necessary in correctly wiring the patient for this procedure, it is important that you also understand the correct operation involved in testing your equipment prior to its use.

The steps followed in ensuring the proper operation of the EKG machine, as well as the time you will need to spend with the patient before the procedure is performed, is referred to as "preliminary steps." As in any skilled task performed by the EKG technician, these preliminary steps are just as important as actually performing the procedure, since their deletion will only hinder the final outcome of the EKG tracing and may ultimately lead to a misdiagnosis of the patient's condition.

To ensure for the proper operation of the EKG machine, always check its function and reliability prior to coming into contact with the patient. In the hospital, this is usually done in the EKG department at the beginning of each work shift, while in the medical office, proper operation of all equipment used on the patient is usually performed on a weekly basis.

In addition to checking your equipment, preliminary steps also include the time spent making your initial contact with the patient. Try to make a practice of always getting your patient in a positive manner, including addressing him or her by name. In the hospital, the greeting and verifying of the patient's name can easily be accomplished by looking at the patient's name band; in the office, checking the patient's name against his or her medical chart may be another effective way of making sure you are performing the procedure on the right person.

During this time you should also spend a few moments explaining the EKG procedure to the patient. This includes answering any questions the patient may have. Remember, however, it is not your responsibility to diagnose or address any questions that have to do with the patient's actual medical condition. This is a job for the physician, and any questions pertaining to diagnosis or treatment must be fielded in such a manner as to not alarm the patient.

Once you have properly explained the procedure and answered any questions the patient may have, your final preliminary step is to make the patient feel as comfortable as possible. This includes providing both physical well-being and emotional security. Placing the patient in a supine position—that is, reclining on his or her back with a pillow under the head—as well as speaking softly and having a gentle touch while connecting the leads will help the patient to relax, thereby making a tense situation much more comfortable. (See Figure 7–1.)

Preliminary Steps for Performing the 3-Channel EKG

The preliminary steps involved in preforming the 3-channel computerized electrocardiogram are quite similar to those required in performing the standard 12-lead EKG. Remember, too, that both units require testing for proper functioning prior to connection to the patient.

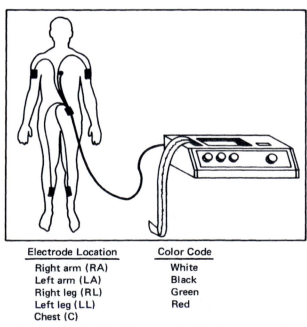

Electrode Location	Color Code
Right arm (RA)	White
Left arm (LA)	Black
Right leg (RL)	Green
Left leg (LL)	Red
Chest (C)	

Figure 7–1 Hooking up the leads correctly.

Before using the E-310 EKG machine, it is advisable that the technician first operate the unit and become familiar with the controls. As the patient cable will not be connected during this preliminary stage, no EKG tracings will be evident during these steps. Instead, what will be noticeable will be the iso-electric, or baseline, and standardization pulse, both of which will appear on the EKG paper. The presence and proper appearance of these markings generally indicate that the unit is functioning properly.

Procedural Steps for Performing the 3-Channel EKG

Once the technician has properly established that the E-310 machine is functioning correctly, and that the patient fully understands the procedure involved in taking the EKG, the technician is ready to begin the procedural steps necessary in performing the EKG. The following guidelines are to be used in performing the procedure on the patient, whether or not the patient is in the hospital or in the medical office:

1. Be sure that the EKG paper has been properly loaded into the machine.
2. Connect the power cord between the E-310 unit and a grounded wall receptacle.
3. Place the power switch in the ON position. Note the functions (LIMB and CHEST sensitivity, SPEED, FILTER, and lead group) that are automatically selected when the unit is turned on.
4. Move the POSITION controls. The styluses should move slowly from the top to the bottom of their respective channels, stopping near the limit lines.
5. Center the styluses with their respective POSITION control.
6. Press the MAN RUN switch. The paper drive should move, and a solid line should be made by each stylus.
7. Press the STOP switch. The paper drive should stop.
8. Ensure that the sensitivities are set to 1, speed at 25 mm/second, filter is out, and 000 is selected.
9. Press the MAN RUN switch. The paper drive should move.
10. Momentarily press the 1 mV switch. The styluses should produce a pulse 10 mm in height. If the deflection of the stylus is more or less than 10 mm, the gain of the unit may require calibration.
11. Examine the leading edge (left side) of the calibration pulse.
12. Press the STOP switch.

PROCEDURAL STEPS FOR PERFORMING THE 12-LEAD EKG

Now that you have completed the preliminary steps necessary for performing the EKG, you are ready to begin the actual steps involved in the EKG procedure. The general procedural steps listed below will help you in completing this task:

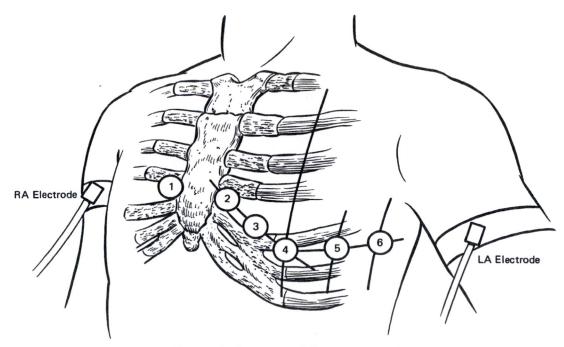

Figure 7–2 Precordial chest lead placement.

1. Prepare the patient's skin by removing any oil, sweat, or scales, using a nonabrasive cleansing agent.
2. Prepare the patient by applying a conductive solution or paste on the patient's arms and legs where the skin will come into contact with the electrode.
3. Apply the electrodes securely to the patient's upper arms and thighs in the same manner as outlined in wiring the patient.
4. Apply the chest electrodes securely.
5. Connect the lead wires to each electrode. *Make sure you use the correct wires.*
6. Plug in the cable that connects the patient to the EKG machine.
7. Check to be certain that the stylus in recording.
8. Start the recording.
9. Turn the machine off and move the chest electrode to another position.
10. Turn on the machine and record the tracing. Repeat step 9 above. You will move the chest electrode to a total of six positions. (See Figure 7–2.)

RECORDING THE STANDARD 12-LEAD EKG

Now that you have completed the necessary preliminary and procedural steps involved in the application of the standard 12-lead EKG, you are ready to begin recording the electrocardiogram. The following guidelines provide the necessary steps for properly recording the standard 12-lead EKG.

1. Assemble all the necessary equipment, including the electrocardiograph machine, the leads, electrodes (sensors), and the electrolyte. Prior to bringing the equipment into the examination room, make sure the room is clean and will be free from any interruptions.

2. Wash your hands.

3. Identify the patient and explain the procedure. Prepare the patient for the examination by asking that he or she remove all clothing from the waist up, including any jewelry that may be around the neck.

4. Ask the patient to lie in a supine position on the examination table. If the patient wishes, a pillow may be placed under the head for comfort during the examination.

5. Drape the patient by exposing only the area in which you will be working. While you are moving the chest leads about, make sure that you provide for the patient's privacy by covering the rest of the chest and the lower half of the body.

6. While explaining the procedure to the patient, ask that he or she remain very still and to relax; any movement may cause unwanted electrical activity on the tracing or (artifacts) and may therefore necessitate redoing the procedure.

7. Place the EKG machine close enough to the patient so that the power cord is away from the examination table and does not run under it.

8. After applying a small amount of electrolyte to the skin, where the sensor will connect, place each of the limb sensors, or electrodes, in position. The two upper sensors should be placed on the upper arms, and the two lower electrodes on the lower legs, with the lead connectors pointed toward the center of the patient's body.

9. If you are using a metal disc chest electrode, you will need to position the chest strap under the patient's left side, with the concave surface of its weighted end of the strap lying against the chest wall.

10. Connect the lead wires to the sensors. Generally, these wires are color-coded, with the abbreviations LA (left arm), LL (left leg), RL (right left), and C (chest) or V (ventricles), which will help you to distinguish one from the other when connecting them to the sensors.

11. Apply the electrolyte to the chest sensors and place it on the first chest lead position (V1). Make sure that the metal disc is held in place by the weighted chest strap.

12. Connect the cable to the sensors. If there is any excess wire, coil it in a loop and fasten it with tape or a band, so that it is out of the way.

13. Position the Lead Selector Switch to ST'D, and center the stylus. Move the Record Switch to 25 mm and check your standardization of the machine by momentarily depressing the ST'D button.

14. Turn the machine to AMP OFF and check whether the amplitude of the ST'D mark is 1 mm on the EKG paper.

15. Center the stylus and run about 10 inches or four to six cycles, of Leads I, II, and III, by moving cycles, of Leads I, II, and III, by moving the Record Switch to RUN (25 mm/second) and turning the Selector Switch to each of the individual positions. If requested by the physician, insert a standardization mark between the T-wave of one EKG cycle and the P-wave of the next.

16. While the watching for any unwanted movement or artifacts, record about 5 to 8 inches of aVR, aVL, and aVF, by turning the Lead Selector to the appropriate position.

17. Record about 5 to 8 inches of each chest lead (V1 to V6), by moving the Lead Selector Switch to its appropriate position. While recording the chest leads, make sure that the machine is turned to the AMP OFF position prior to moving and recording any of the chest leads.

18. Complete the recording by positioning the Lead Selector Switch back to ST'D and running off approximately 12 inches. Make sure to properly identify the tracing with the patient's name, the date and time of the recording, and your initials.

19. Turn the machine OFF, unplug the power cord, and disconnect the lead wires. Remove the sensors and rubber strap from the patient, making sure to clean off any leftover electrolyte from the patient's skin.

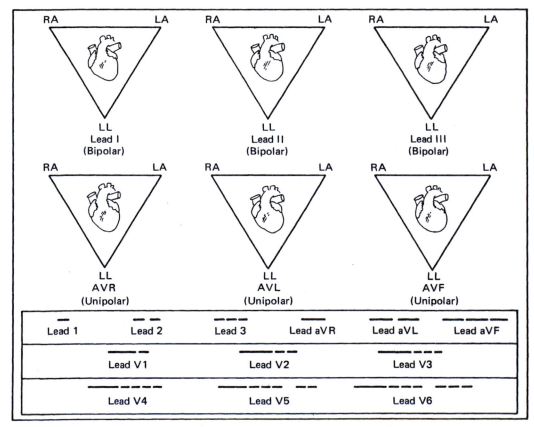

Figure 7–3 Standard leads and marking codes.

20. Help the patient off the examination table and assist as needed.
21. Clean and return the equipment according to the policy of the hospital or office.
22. Wash your hands.
23. Record the procedure in the patient's chart, making sure to put down both the date and time of the recording. (See Figures 7–3 and 7–4.)

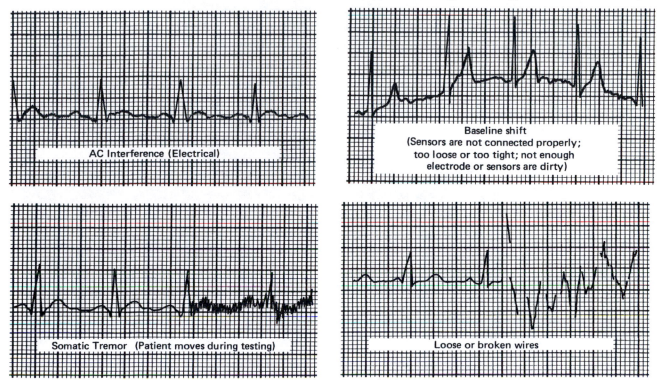

Figure 7–4   Types of artifacts.

RECORDING THE 3-CHANNEL COMPUTERIZED EKG

The main difference between recording the electrocardiogram on the 3-channel computerized EKG machine versus the standard 12-lead machine is that the computerized machine makes the recording a great deal easier. This is because the majority of the steps outlined in the standard 12-lead recording are completed automatically on the computerized unit. However, when required to record the tracing on the computerized machine, the following guidelines will be helpful for your preliminary recording:

1. Assemble your necessary equipment.
2. Wash your hands.
3. Identify the patient and explain the procedure.
4. Begin the auto sequence operation:
   a. Connect the patient cable to both the patient and to the unit.

b. Place the POWER switch in the ON position.

c. If desired, make sensitivity, speed, or filter changes. Remember, any changes to the sensitivity, speed, or filter may not be made during an auto sequence.

d. Press the AUTO RUN switch.

e. The paper will be queued to the correct point and the unit will automatically record each lead group and stop when the sequence has been completed. Pressing the STOP switch during this mode will terminate the auto sequence, thereby allowing a different selection to be made.

To perform a manual sequence operation using the 3-channel computerized unit, the following guidelines should be followed:

1. Connect the patient cable to both the ptaient and to the unit.
2. Place the POWER switch in the ON position.
3. If necessary, make the appropriate sensitivity, speed, or filter changes.
4. Press the LEAD SELECT switch of the desired lead group
5. Press the MAN RUN switch.
6. The selected lead group will be recorded until a new lead group is selected, or when the AUTO RUN or STOP switch is pressed, or when the unit is turned off.

MOUNTING THE EKG TRACING

The technique for properly mounting the EKG tracing is just as important as the skills involved in recording it. The purpose of mounting the tracing is to provide the physician with a sharp, concise pictorial "history" of what the patient's heart is doing; the tracing can then be inserted into the patient's medical chart for future use.

To mount the electrocardiogram properly, the EKG technician should follow the guidelines listed here:

1. Assemble the necessary equipment. This will include an EKG ruler, the electrocardiogram tracing that had previously been run, an EKG mount, and a pair of scissors.
2. Wash your hands.
3. Label the EKG tracing with the correct information, including the patient's name, the date and time the tracing was completed, the patient's age, his or address if required, and the physician's name.
4. Unroll the EKG tracing carefully so as to avoid any possible scratches on the paper. Never, under any circumstances, fold EKG paper; this can leave bend marks, making interpretation of the tracing almost impossible.
5. Locate Lead I. Find the correct ST'D mark, making sure it is centered between the complexes. Once Lead I has been located, position the

ruler so that the ST'D is centered in the middle of the length required for Lead I. Use a pen, pencil, or fingernail to make a small mark on the upper margin at each end of the required length. Gently place the ruler vertically along the end of the required length and hold it securely so that you can tear the paper evenly. Slip the ruler into the Lead I slot, making sure it is open and loose enough to mount the tracing into it. Remove the protective cover or expose the tape or sticky surface on self-stick mounts. Fold approximately one-quarter inch of the paper over the end of the ruler, making sure to hold the strip in place while sliding it into the Lead I area on the slot mount. If using self-stick mounts, position the recording and press gently to the sticky surface. Check to make sure the recording is firmly attached to the mount. On slot mounts, hold the strip in place gently while moving the ruler. Check to ensure that the strip is mounted neatly, the ST'D is centered and correct, and the complexes are clear.

6. Repeat the same steps as in step 5 above, for the remaining leads. Use the marked areas on the EKG ruler to determine the length of each lead.

7. Recheck the entire mount to assure it is neat, mounted correctly, and has the proper standards in each lead.

8. Replace all equipment according to the hospital or office policy.

9. Wash your hands.

REVIEW QUESTIONS

Directions: For the questions below, give the answers you believe are most
correct:

1. What is the purpose of recording an electrocardiogram?

2. The electrocardiogram is primarily used as a _____

   _____ in determining the status of the patient's heart.

3. Heart and cardiovascular diseases affect more than _____ million Americans each year.

4. Give at least one reason the physician might order an electrocardiogram.

5. Define what is mean by "preliminary steps" for performing an electrocardiogram:

6. How many tasks are involved in the preliminary steps pertaining to recording an electrocardiogram?

7. How many precordial chest leads are used in recording to standard 12-lead
   electrocardiogram?

8. You should always record the _____ and _____

   _____ of the electrocardiogram recording.

9. Identify the four basic types of artifacts seen on an electrocardiogram
   recording:

   (a) _____

   (b) _____

   (c) _____

   (d) _____

10. What is the main difference between recording the EKG tracing on a stan-
    dard 12-lead EKG machine and a computerized machine?

11. The purpose of mounting the electrocardiogram is to provide the physician

    with a pictorial _____ of the patient's heart.

Basic EKG Interpretation: Recognizing Abnormal Electrocardiograms

8

TERMINAL OBJECTIVE

To provide the student with a basic understanding of EKG interpretation so as to recognize abnormal electrocardiograms.

COMPETENCY OBJECTIVES

Upon completion of this chapter, the student will be able to

1. Identify the four elements involved in EKG interpretation.
2. Discuss the various components of the cardiac cycle.
3. Explain how to recognize an abnormal electrocardiogram.
4. Discuss arrhythmias and identify how to interpret arrhythmias of the SA node, sinus tachycardia, sinus arrest, wandering pacemaker, and sinus bradycardia.
5. Discuss atrial tachycardias and explain how to identify them on an EKG tracing.
6. Discuss atrial flutter and explain how to identify it on an EKG tracing.
7. Discuss atrial fibrillation and explain how to identify it on an EKG tracing.
8. Describe what occurs during premature atrial contractions.
9. Discuss ventricular arrhythmias and know how to recognize and interpret ventricular fibrillation, ventricular flutter, and ventricular asystole.
10. Discuss a right and left bundle branch block and explain how they can be identified on the EKG tracing.
11. Discuss a first- and second-degree A-V block and explain how they can be identified on the EKG tracing.
12. Discuss premature ventricular contractions and explain how to recognize and identify them on the EKG tracing.

BASIC INTERPRETATION

Before we can begin to discuss some of the more frequently seen abnormal electrocardiograms and the arrhythmias caused by the heart, which they indicate, it is important that we first examine the basic components that we look for on the abnormal electrocardiogram. We refer to this examination of the EKG tracing as *basic interpretation.*

There are four elements that we look at when performing basic EKG interpretation. These are the rate, rhythm, conduction, and configuration of each of the segments of the EKG strip.

Rate

Rate stands for the number of pulse rates and heartbeats per minute. It may be calculated either by using the apex of the wave or the initial upstroke of the wave. To calculate the rate, the EKG technician counts the number of small squares (1 mm × 1 mm) between the R-wave (to get the vertical rate) or between the P-waves (to get the atrial rate). That number is then divided into 1,500*, with the sum given as the accurate heart rate.

A second way to calculate the heart rate is to count the large squares (5 mm × 5 mm) between the R-wave of one cycle to the R-wave of the next cycle and then divide that number by 300.*

The technician may use a third way to calculate the heart rate: counting the number of cardiac cycles in 6 seconds and multiplying that number by 10. Considered the least accurate of all three methods, it is the easiest to use during tachycardia.

Rhythm

Rhythm pertains to the regularity of the heartbeats. Usually a glance is enough to determine whether the rhythm is regular or irregular; however, to be more accurate, the technician should measure with the caliper or ruler in order to see if the distance between each R-wave is equal to the next.

Conduction

Conduction refers to the time it takes for the impulse originating at the SA node to stimulate ventricular contraction. It is found by measuring the P-R interval and the QRS duration.

*Preset number used to determine rates.

106

Configuration

Configuration and the location of the waves on the EKG tracing will tell the technician about the extent and location of any myocardial damage. In order to determine the configuration, the technician should ask the following questions: (1) Are the waves similar in shape and size? (2) Do the waves point in the same direction? and (3) Are the waves upright, inverted, or diphasic? (See Figure 8–1.)

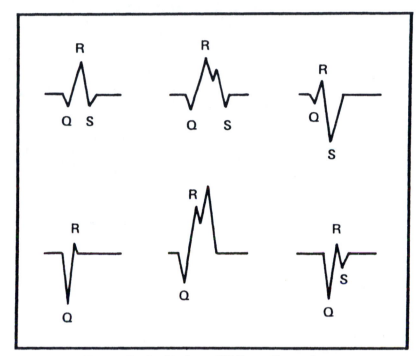

Figure 8–1 Various QRS configurations.

EKG INTERPRETATION AND THE CARDIAC CYCLE

A single cardiac cycle of the electrical activity as recorded on an EKG tracing or strip gives information that may appear in a typical normal lead. Any variations could indicate abnormalities.

Each cardiac cycle is indicative of certain actions occurring in the heart. And each one of these actions is represented by a specific feature found on the EKG tracing. These include the "P-wave," "P-R interval," "QRS-complex," "S-T segment," "T-wave," "U-wave," and the "Q-T duration."

The P-Wave

A P-wave represents the contraction of the atria; normally, it should not exceed more than 0.11 seconds. It will appear upright in leads 1, 2, and aVf, and varies in leads 3, aV1, and V1 through V6.

The P-R Interval

The P-R interval represents how long it has taken the electrical impulse to travel from the SA node to the bundle of His. Normally it should take anywhere from 0.12 to 0.20 seconds and is best measured from the beginning of the P-wave to the beginning of the QRS-complex, and then multiplied by 0.04. (See Figure 8–2.)

The QRS Duration

The QRS duration represents the spread of impulse through the ventricular muscle, or what we refer to as *depolarization*. Normally it should take from 0.05 to 0.11 seconds and is measured from the beginning of the Q to the S, and then multiplied by 0.04. Any measurement over 0.12 seconds may be an indication of an abnormal ventricular conduction or bundle branch block, or a ventricular arrhythmia.

The S-T Segment

The S-T segment represents the resting period between depolarization and repolarization. Normally it is viewed as a flat isoelectric line, and is measured from the beginning of the S to the beginning of the T-wave. To determine if the S-T segment is elevated or depressed, the technician should place the straight edge of a paper along the baseline. Above the line represents an elevation, and below the line represents a depression.

The T-Wave

The T-wave represents the recovery period of the ventricles. Normally all T-waves should be the same size and shape throughout the strip, should point in the same direction as the QRS-complexes, and are measured from the beginning to the end of each T-wave.

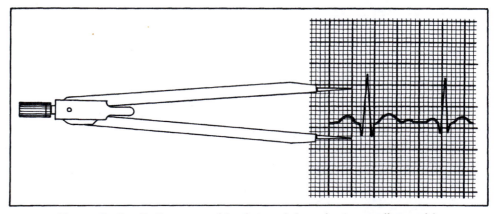

Figure 8–2   Calipers used in determining electrocardiographic intervals.

The U-Wave

This is a small wave, sometimes seen following the T-wave, and often when a patient has a potassium deficiency.

The Q-T Interval

The Q-T interval is responsible for giving the physician a better picture of the total ventricular activity of the heart. It is measured from the *Q* to the end of the T-wave, and often varies with the heart rate, sex, and age of the patient. It may also lengthen with the presence of congestive heart failure and myocardial infarction. (See Figures 8–3, 8–4.)

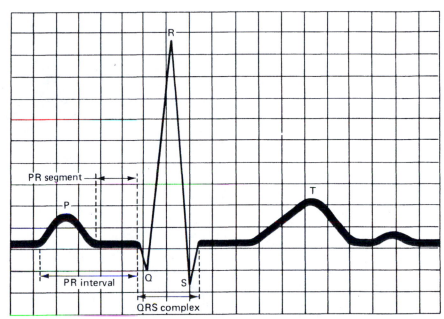

Figure 8–3   The EKG complex.

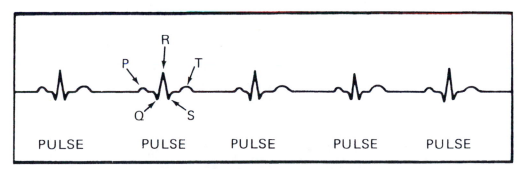

Figure 8–4   Typical EKG rhythm strip. In a healthy heart, each cardiac cycle would be expected to correlate with the patient's individual pulse beats. (Reprinted with permission from *Basic Arrhythmias, 3/E* by Gail Walraven, Prentice Hall, Inc., Englewood Cliffs, NJ 07632.)

RECOGNIZING ABNORMAL ELECTROCARDIOGRAMS

Although many different types of abnormal and irregular heartbeats may surface on the electrocardiogram tracing, we will concentrate on the more frequently seen abnormalities. The most important point the EKG technician should be aware of is that, anytime the tracing appears to show any irregular peculiarities or deviations from what is considered the "normal" EKG recording, these changes must be reported immediately, so that the patient's health is not jeopardized and that treatment may be started without delay. (See Figure 8–5.)

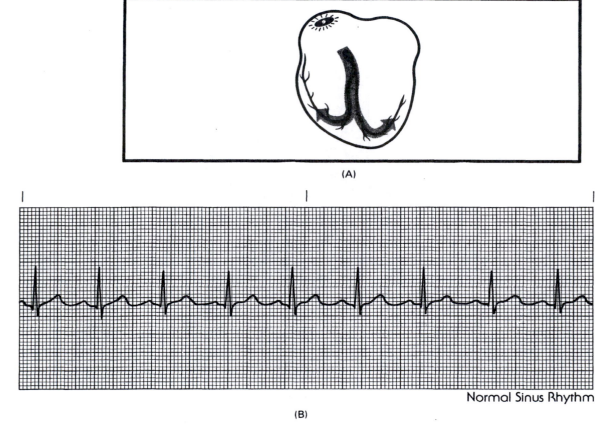

(A)

Normal Sinus Rhythm

(B)

Figure 8–5   (A) Normal sinus rhythm; (B) EKG strip showing normal sinus rhythm. (Reprinted with permission from *Basic Arrhythmias, 3/E* by Gail Walraven, Prentice Hall, Inc., Englewood Cliffs, NJ 07632.)

UNDERSTANDING ARRHYTHMIAS

A normal heartbeat—that is, one ranging from 60 to 100 beats per minute—is called *normal sinus rhythm*. When this sinus rhythm begins to deviate, causing abnormally decreased or increased beats to occur, a chain reaction results, triggering what is known as an *arrhythmia*.

An arrhythmia is a term generally used to describe all forms of abnormalities, including disturbances in the rate, rhythm, and conduction within the cardiac rhythm of the heart. Some of the more typical irregularities that cause cardiac arrhythmias include sinus bradycardia; atrial flutter; right and left bundle branch blocks; sinus tachycardia; premature atrial contractions; atrial fibrillation; first-, second-, and third-degree heart block; ventricular tachycardia; premature ventricular contractions; ventricular fibrillation, and the most fatal of all arrhythmias, ventricular asystole.

The majority of cardiac arrhythmias are classified according to their effect upon the anatomical structure of the heart. They include arrhythmias of the sinoatrial or SA node, atrial tachycardias, premature atrial contractions, and ventricular arrhythmias.

ARRHYTHMIAS OF THE SA NODE

Arrhythmias originating in the sinoatrial, or SA node, are considered the least dangerous of all arrhythmias. The most common of these include sinus bradycardia, sinus tachycardia, sinus arrest, and a wandering pacemaker.

Sinus Bradycardia

Sinus bradycardia is characterized as a sinus rate that falls below 60 beats per minute, with all impulses still originating from the SA node. This condition may be found in persons whose health is normal, especially

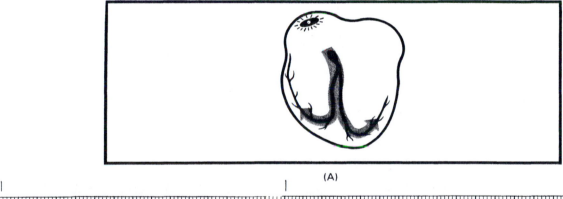

(A)

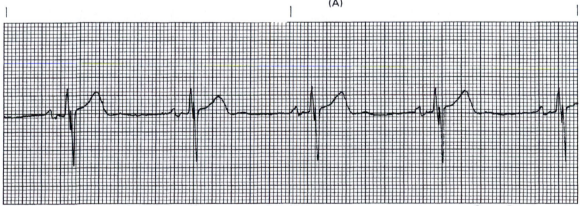

Sinus Bradycardia

(B)

Figure 8-6   (A) Sinus bradycardia; (B) EKG strip showing sinus bradycardia. (Reprinted with permission from *Basic Arrhythmias, 3/E* by Gail Walraven, Prentice Hall, Inc., Englewood Cliffs, NJ 07632.)

athletes, who have an enlarged heart because of the use of excessive exercise. Sinus bradycardia may also be found as an underlying heart disease, as in the case of a myocardial infarction. (See Figure 8–6.)

Sinus Tachycardia

Sinus tachycardia is just the opposite of sinus bradycardia—that is, in this condition the sinus rate exceeds the norm, usually ranging between 100 to 160 beats per minute. It is commonly seen in normal, healthy people and may be related to anxiety or strenuous exercise. (See Figure 8–7.)

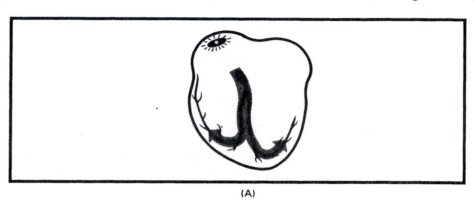

(A)

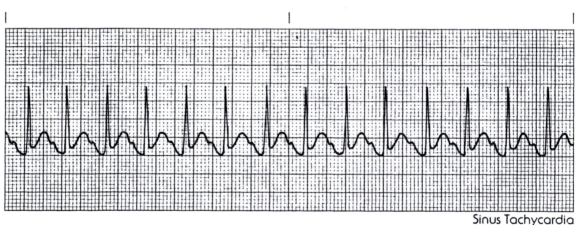

Sinus Tachycardia

(B)

Figure 8–7 (A) Sinus tachycardia; (B) EKG strip showing sinus tachycardia. (Reprinted with permission from *Basic Arrhythmias, 3/E* by Gail Walraven, Prentice Hall, Inc., Englewood Cliffs, NJ 07632.)

Sinus Arrest

Occasionally the SA node will fail momentarily and will not initiate an impulse. This may be due to an increased vagal stimulation, such as overeating, excessive consumption of coffee or cigarettes, pharyngeal massage, or deep inspiration. If this momentary stopping of the impulse does occur, sinus arrest may result. (See Figure 8–8.)

During sinus arrest, there is a literal atrial standstill, in which the atria are not stimulated to contract, thereby causing no atrial activity. What results in the EKG tracing are long pauses in which beats are

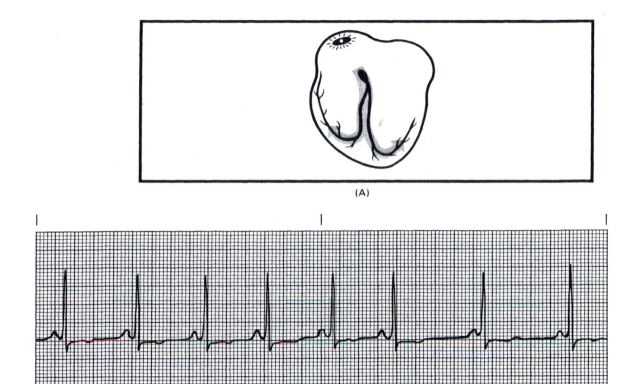

(A)

Sinus Arrhythmia

(B)

Figure 8-8 (A) Sinus arrhythmia; (B) EKG strip showing sinus arrhythmia. (Reprinted with permission from *Basic Arrhythmias, 3/E* by Gail Walraven, Prentice Hall, Inc., Englewood Cliffs, NJ 07632.)

dropped. In the normal sinus rhythm tracing, the P-wave and QRS-complex appear normal; however, in the sinus arrest EKG strip, there is no P-wave, and the pause, appearing as a straight line, is followed by the QRS-complex.

Wandering Pacemaker

The fourth type of arrhythmia found in the SA node is referred to as a *wandering pacemaker*. It is a confusing arrhythmia because the site of the impulse shifts. Sometimes the beats originate in the SA node; other times they occur in the AV node or an irritable atrial focus. (See Figure 8-9.)

Because the pacemaker site shifts, the P-waves vary in configuration and direction and the P-R intervals vary in length. The ventricular rhythms can also vary slightly.

A wandering pacemaker may be caused by irritated atrial tissues stemming from rheumatic carditis or infection, or an excessive buildup of the heart medication digitalis. Ironically, despite its unusual configuration, wandering pacemaker is rarely considered dangerous or life-threatening.

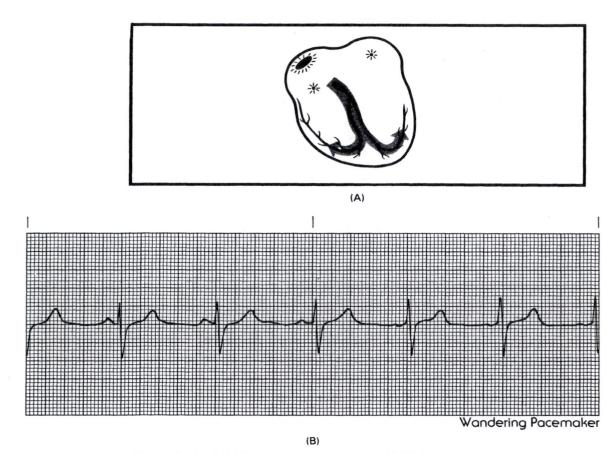

(A)

Wandering Pacemaker

(B)

Figure 8–9   (A) Wandering pacemaker; (B) EKG strip showing wandering pacemaker. (Reprinted with permission from *Basic Arrhythmias*, *3/E* by Gail Walraven, Prentice Hall, Inc., Englewood Cliffs, NJ 07632.)

ATRIAL TACHYCARDIAS

The second group of arrhythmias are referred to as *atrial tachycardias*. There are three different types of atrial tachycardias, each with a different mechanism, and all three originate from an atrial ectopic foci and have rates in excess of 160 beats per minute. (See Figure 8–10.)

Paroxysmal Atrial Tachycardia (PAT)

Paroxysmal atrial tachycardias, or what we refer to as PATs, may occur in normal, healthy persons. However, when they strike in cardiac patients, or someone who is critically ill, they can be considered a forerunner to a very serious ventricular arrhythmia.

A PAT is a very rapid regular heartbeat that begins suddenly and usually has been preceded by frequent PACs, or premature atrial contractions. (See discussion later in chapter.) In some cases, the tachycardia is brief, while at other times it can last for hours.

If the physician believes the patient is suffering from PATs, he or she will usually try one of two procedures to try to slow down the rate.

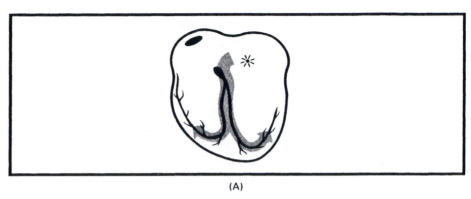

(A)

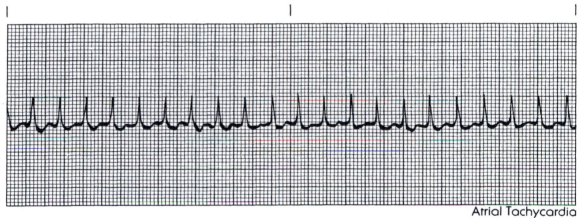

Atrial Tachycardia

(B)

Figure 8-10 (A) Atrial tachycardia; (B) EKG strip showing atrial tachycardia. (Reprinted with permission from *Basic Arrhythmias, 3/E* by Gail Walraven, Prentice Hall, Inc., Englewood Cliffs, NJ 07632.)

The first, called Valsalva's maneuver, involves having the patient take deep breaths and bearing down, or "pushing" the breaths out. The second involves the physician stimulating the carotid artery by using pressure. Both methods stimulate the vagus nerve and therefore slow down the impulse production, causing atrial standstill. This allows the SA node to reestablish itself as the pacemaker.

Atrial Flutter

A second type of atrial tachycardia is called *atrial flutter*. It is oftentimes misdiagnosed as a PAT, since the impulse comes from an atrial ectopic focus. It differs from the tachycardia in that, if the SA node has no control of the impulse and the atria are in control, the atria tend to beat about 300 beats per minute.

In patients suffering from atrial flutter, the actual atrial rates range from 220 to 350 beats per minute, while the ventricles beat approximately 75 beats per minute. Interestingly enough, in most cases of atrial flutter the rhythm of the ventricles is almost always regular.

Most patients afflicted with atrial flutter respond well to digitalis, which may or may not be given in combination with the drug Inderal, to obtain quicker results.

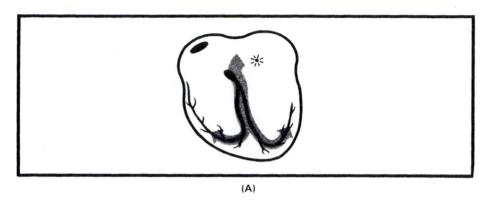

(A)

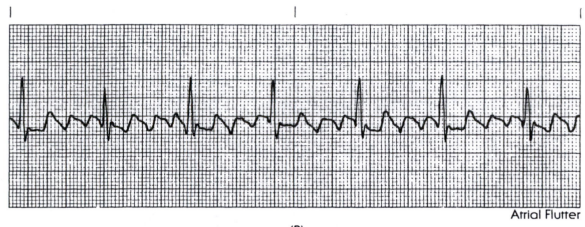

Atrial Flutter

(B)

Figure 8–11 (A) Atrial flutter; (B) EKG strip showing atrial flutter. (Reprinted with permission from *Basic Arrhythmias, 3/E* by Gail Walraven, Prentice Hall, Inc., Englewood Cliffs, NJ 07632.)

Atrial flutter is seen on the EKG tracing as a merging together of both the T-wave and the P-wave, in order to form a "sawtooth" flutter wave. The QRS-complex usually narrows and the flutter waves are more uniform in width. (See Figure 8–11.)

Atrial Fibrillation

The third type of atrial tachycardia, called *atrial fibrillation*, is generally easily recognized, because of its grossly irregular ventricular rhythm. As with the other two atrial arrhythmias, in atrial fibrillation the impulse originates in an atrial ectopic area, thereby creating a chaotic baseline.

In fibrillation, the flutter waves are not uniform and vary in shape and width. They can "fire" as high as 500 beats per minute, causing the P-R interval also to be very irregular.

Patients admitted to the hospital with the diagnosis of atrial fibrillation are usually treated with medications that control the heart rhythm, thus bringing the fibrillation back to a normal sinus rhythm. Therefore, no dramatic treatment is generally necessary. (See Figure 8–12.)

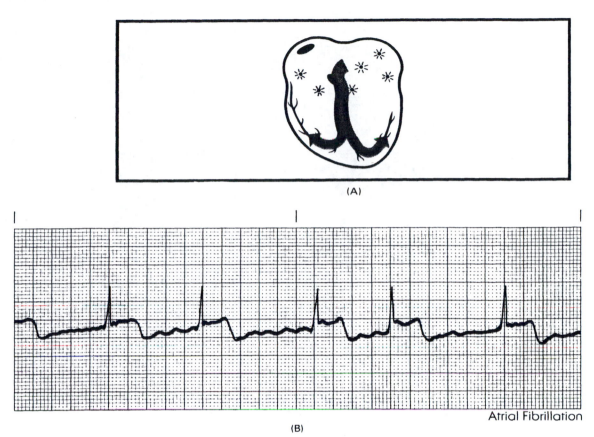

(A)

Atrial Fibrillation

(B)

Figure 8-12   (A) Atrial fibrillation; (B) EKG strip showing atrial fibrillation. (Reprinted with permission from *Basic Arrhythmias, 3/E* by Gail Walraven, Prentice Hall, Inc., Englewood Cliffs, NJ 07632.)

PREMATURE ATRIAL CONTRACTIONS (PACs)

Premature atrial contractions (PACs) originate from an atrial ectopic focus, thereby producing an abnormal P-wave earlier than expected. Because the impulse does not originate in the SA node, this arrhythmia may appear like other P-waves in the same lead.

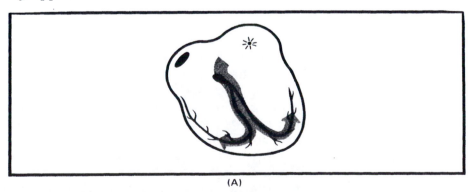

(A)

Figure 8-13   (A) Premature atrial contraction (PAC); (Reprinted with permission from *Basic Arrhythmias, 3/E* by Gail Walraven, Prentice Hall, Inc., Englewood Cliffs, NJ 07632.)

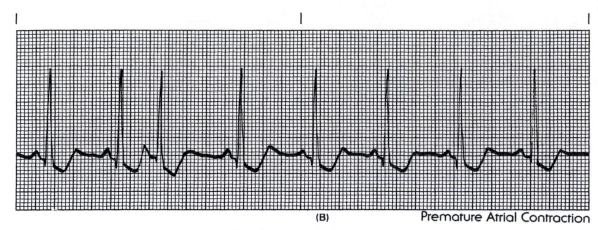

(B)   Premature Atrial Contraction

Figure 8–13 (cont.) (B) EKG strip showing premature atrial contractions. (Reprinted with permission from *Basic Arrhythmias, 3/E* by Gail Walraven, Prentice Hall, Inc., Englewood Cliffs, NJ 07632.)

In the EKG tracing, PACs generally portray an abnormal P-wave configuration, such as being flat, slurred, notched, inverted, or wide. The P-R interval of the premature beat also appears shorter than normal, depending upon the location of the P-wave. The pause following the premature beat does not occur at the normal time, since the SA timing was disturbed. And the QRS-complex, interestingly enough, usually appears normal. (See Figure 8–13.)

VENTRICULAR ARRHYTHMIAS

Ventricular arrhythmias are almost always considered serious and usually occur suddenly, oftentimes resulting in rapid death despite vigorous treatment. Those included in this category include premature ventricular contractions, ventricular tachycardia, ventricular fibrillation, ventricular flutter, ventricular asystole, right and left bundle branch blocks, and first-, second-, and third-degree A-V blocks.

Premature Ventricular Contraction (PVC)

Premature ventricular contractions originate in the ectopic focus of the ventricular myocardium. While they may occur in seemingly healthy persons, they are most often seen when the heart is diseased or injured.

On the EKG tracing, the PVC appears with a wide, bizarre-shaped QRS-complex, with no preceeding P-wave. Often, the QRS points in the opposite direction from the patient's normal QRS-complex. The T-wave that follows is also wider and larger and usually points in the opposite direction from the QRS-complex.

During premature ventricular contractions the ventricles are stimulated prematurely and therefore contract before the expected time. And their seriousness is determined not only by how often they occur but also by how close they are to the T-wave of the preceding beat.

PVCs tend to surface in patients with slow heart rates and are often associated with poor cardiac output. (See Figures 8–14 through 8–22.)

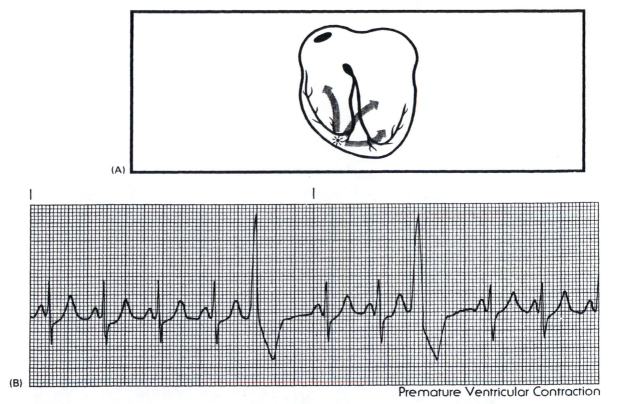

(A)

(B)

Premature Ventricular Contraction

Figure 8-14 (A) Premature ventricular contraction (PVC); (B) EKG strip showing premature ventricular contraction. (Reprinted with permission from *Basic Arrhythmias, 3/E* by Gail Walraven, Prentice Hall, Inc., Englewood Cliffs, NJ 07632.)

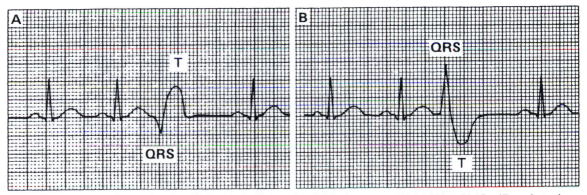

Figure 8-15 EKG strip showing T-wave configuration in a PVC. (Reprinted with permission from *Basic Arrhythmias, 3/E* by Gail Walraven, Prentice Hall, Inc., Englewood Cliffs, NJ 07632.)

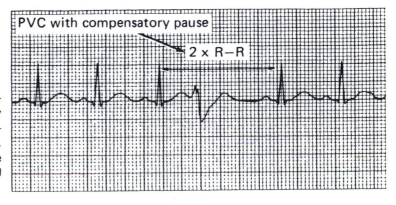

Figure 8-16 EKG strip showing a PVC with a compensatory pause. (Reprinted with permission from *Basic Arrhythmias, 3/E* by Gail Walraven, Prentice Hall, Inc., Englewood Cliffs, NJ 07632.)

119

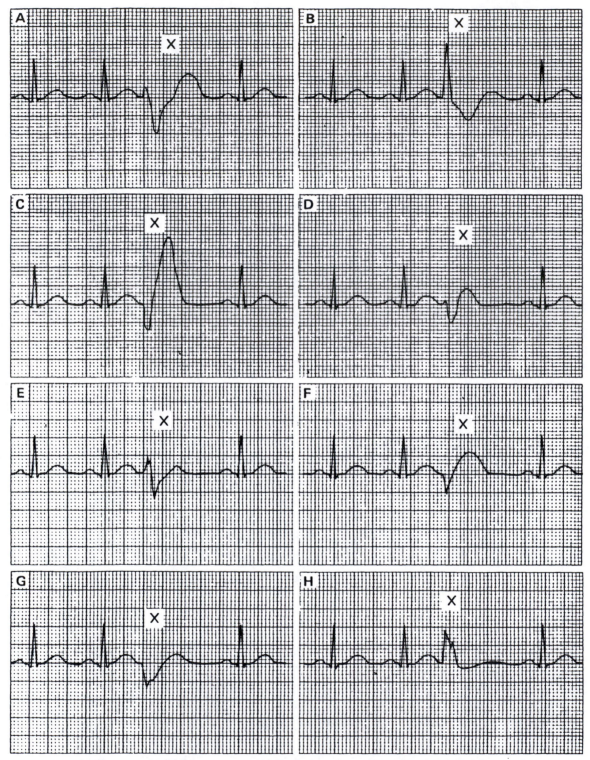

Figure 8-17   EKG strips showing typical PVC configurations. (Reprinted with permission from *Basic Arrhythmias, 3/E* by Gail Walraven, Prentice Hall, Inc., Englewood Cliffs, NJ 07632.)

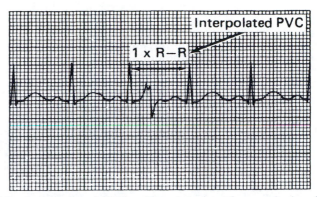

Figure 8–18   Interpolated PVCs. (Reprinted with permission from *Basic Arrhythmias, 3/E* by Gail Walraven, Prentice Hall, Inc., Englewood Cliffs, NJ 07632.)

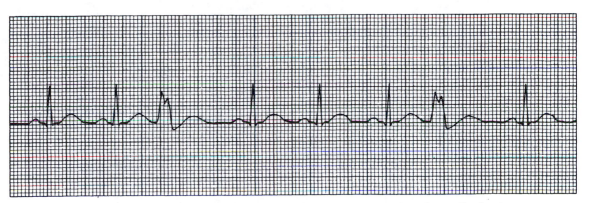

Figure 8–19   Unifocal PVCs. (Reprinted with permission from *Basic Arrhythmias, 3/E* by Gail Walraven, Prentice Hall, Inc., Englewood Cliffs, NJ 07632.)

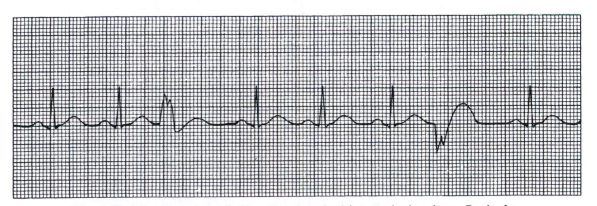

Figure 8–20   Multifocal PVCs. (Reprinted with permission from *Basic Arrhythmias, 3/E* by Gail Walraven, Prentice Hall, Inc., Englewood Cliffs, NJ 07632.)

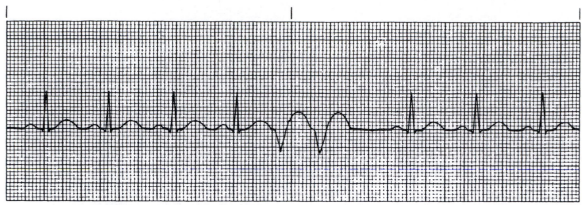

Figure 8-21 PVCs occurring in pairs. (Reprinted with permission from *Basic Arrhythmias, 3/E* by Gail Walraven, Prentice Hall, Inc., Englewood Cliffs, NJ 07632.)

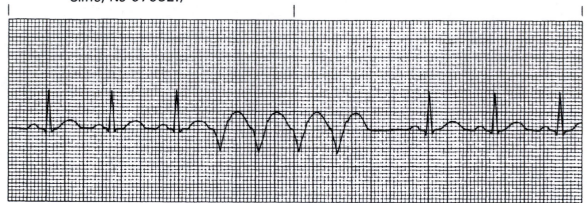

Figure 8-22 PVCs occurring in a "run." (Reprinted with permission from *Basic Arrhythmias, 3/E* by Gail Walraven, Prentice Hall, Inc., Englewood Cliffs, NJ 07632.)

Ventricular Tachycardia

On the EKG tracing, ventricular tachycardia is most often identified by its wide, uniform QRS-complex and a regular rhythm. Because most patients cannot tolerate high ventricular rates for long periods of time, they must be treated immediately with intravenous lidocaine. Oftentimes cardio shock is used in order to revert the heart back to a normal sinus rhythm. (See Figure 8-23.)

Ventricular Fibrillation (V-Fib)

Ventricular fibrillation is created by stimuli from many ventricular ectopic foci, causing a chaotic twitching of the ventricles. Because there are so many ventricular ectopic foci "firing" at once, each of which discharging only a small area of the ventricle, this results in an ineffective pumping action occurring in the ventricles.

Ventricular fibrillation is considered a life-threatening emergency. There is no characteristic pattern seen on the EKG tracing, and if the technician is unable to recognize any repetition of pattern or regularity, then he or she is probably dealing with V-Fib. (See Figure 8-24.)

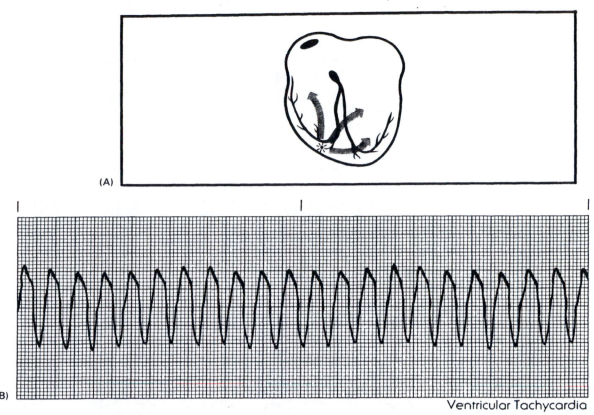

(A)

(B) Ventricular Tachycardia

Figure 8-23 (A) Ventricular tachycardia; (B) EKG strip showing ventricular tachycardia. (Reprinted with permission from *Basic Arrhythmias, 3/E* by Gail Walraven, Prentice Hall, Inc., Englewood Cliffs, NJ 07632.)

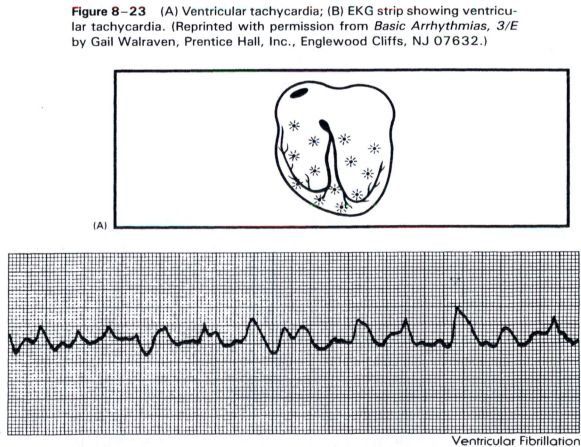

(A)

(B) Ventricular Fibrillation

Figure 8-24 (A) Ventricular fibrillation; (B) EKG strip showing ventricular fibrillation. (Reprinted with permission from *Basic Arrhythmias, 3/E* by Gail Walraven, Prentice Hall, Inc., Englewood Cliffs, NJ 07632.)

Ventricular Flutter

This condition is preceded by a single ventricular ecoptic focus firing at a rate of 200 to 300 times per minute. There is also a noticeable "smooth" wave appearance on the EKG tracing.

Ventricular flutter is characterized by an extremely fast rate and is considered a highly dangerous condition, deteriorating quickly into deadly arrhythmias.

Ventricular Asystole

Of all the cardiac emergencies, asystole, or ventricular standstill, is considered to strike the greatest fear among nurses. It is always life-threatening; however, it does not always have to be fatal.

Asystole means the absence of contraction. The heart does not beat and its appearance on the EKG tracing is noted as a "straight line." It is commonly caused as a direct result of hypoxia, or impaired respiratory function; however, it can also be caused from a drug overdose. (See Figure 8–25.)

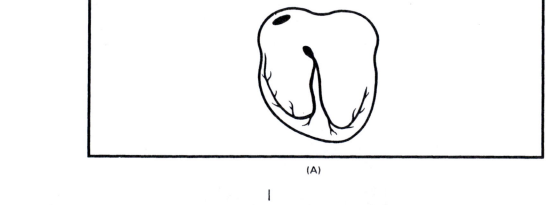

(A)

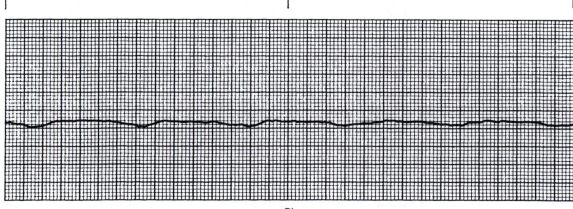

(B)

Figure 8–25   (A) Ventricular asystole; (B) EKG strip showing ventricular asystole. (Reprinted with permission from *Basic Arrhythmias, 3/E* by Gail Walraven, Prentice Hall, Inc., Englewood Cliffs, NJ 07632.)

Right and Left Bundle Branch Blocks

A right bundle branch block is usually accompanied by sinus tachycardia. In the EKG tracing, the P-Wave is not distinct; therefore it may resemble ventricular tachycardia.

In a left bundle branch block, the rhythm may resemble ventricular tachycardia if there is sinus tachycardia, and atrial activity, such as when the P-wave precedes a QRS-complex (a very rare occurrence).

First- and Second-Degree A-V Block

A first-degree heart block is defined as a complete heart block, in which case the atria and ventricles are seen to be beating independently. There is no fixed relationship between the P-waves and the QRS-complexes.

A second-degree block exists when a P-wave is not followed by a QRS-complex. In one type of second-degree A-V block, called the Wenckebach phenomenon, there is a progressive prolongation of the P-R interval until finally a P-wave fails to conduct to the ventricles. (See Figure 8–26.)

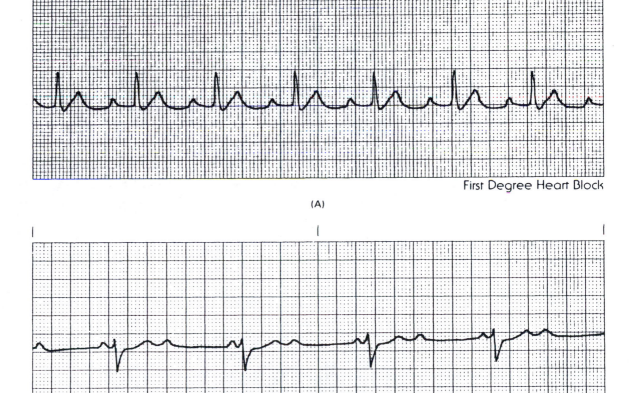

First Degree Heart Block

(A)

Classical Second Degree Heart Block

(B)

Figure 8–26 Heart blocks: (A) first-degree heart block; (B) second-degree heart block; (Reprinted with permission from *Basic Arrhythmias*, *3/E* by Gail Walraven, Prentice Hall, Inc., Englewood Cliffs, NJ 07632.)

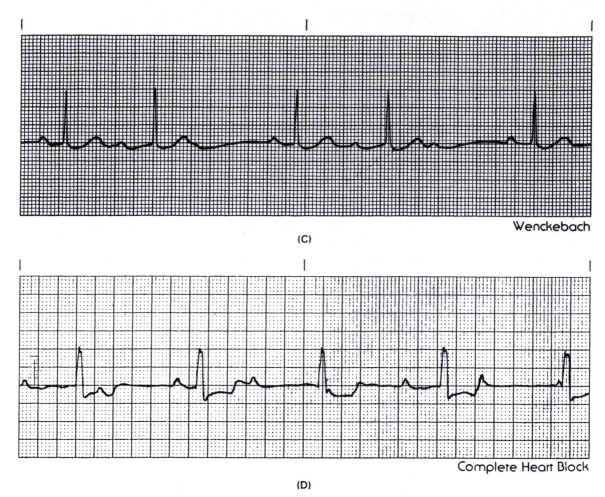

Wenckebach

(C)

Complete Heart Block

(D)

Figure 8-26 (*cont.*) (C) Wenckebach second-degree heart block; (D) complete heart block. (Reprinted with permission from *Basic Arrhythmias, 3/E* by Gail Walraven, Prentice Hall, Inc., Englewood Cliffs, NJ 07632.)

REVIEW QUESTIONS

Directions: For the questions below, give the answers you believe are most correct:

1. How many elements are involved in EKG interpretation?

2. List the elements of EKG interpretation:

3. What does a *P-wave* represent?

4. What does the *P-R interval* represent?

5. What does the *QRS duration* represent?

6. What does the *S-T segment* represent?

7. What does the *T-wave* represent?

8. When is the U-wave most often seen and where is it located?

9. What is the range for a normal, healthy adult heartbeat?

10. Define bradycardia:

11. Define tachycardia:

12. Define arrhythmia:

13. What occurs during sinus arrest?

14. Identify at least one atrial tachycardia condition:

15. Where does a *PAC* originate from and how is it interpreted?

16. Give at least one example of a ventricular arrhythmia:

17. What causes *ventricular fibrillation* and what occurs in the ventricles during its occurrence?

18. How is *ventricular tachycardia* identified on the EKG tracing?

19. What is *ventricular asystole,* and how is it identified on the EKG tracing?

20. Label the waves below:

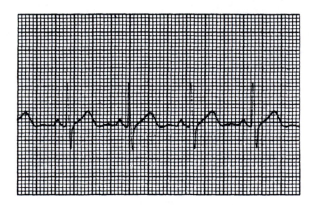

(Reprinted with permission from *Basic Arrhythmias, 3/E* by Gail Walraven, Prentice Hall, Inc., Englewood Cliffs, NJ 07632.)

21. Label the intervals and seconds of each tracing below:

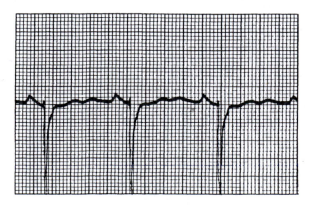

(Reprinted with permission from *Basic Arrhythmias, 3/E* by Gail Walraven, Prentice Hall, Inc., Englewood Cliffs, NJ 07632.)

PRI: _____ seconds
QRS: _____ seconds

22. Fill in the information below for the *atrial rhythm:*

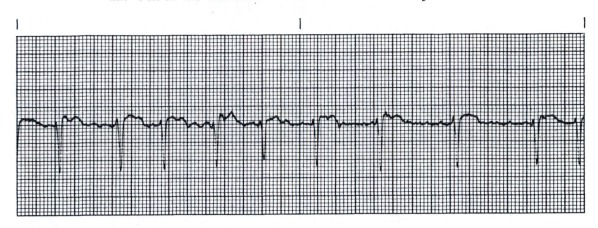

(Reprinted with permission from *Basic Arrhythmias, 3/E* by Gail Walraven,
Prentice Hall, Inc., Englewood Cliffs, NJ 07632.)

Regularity: _____
Rate: _____
P Waves: _____
PRI: _____
QRS: _____
Interp: _____

23. Fill in the information below for a *ventricular rhythm:*

(Reprinted with permission from *Basic Arrhythmias, 3/E* by Gail Walraven,
Prentice Hall, Inc., Englewood Cliffs, NJ 07632.)

Regularity: _____
Rate: _____
P Waves: _____
PRI: _____
QRS: _____
Interp: _____

24. Fill in the information below for a *heart block:*

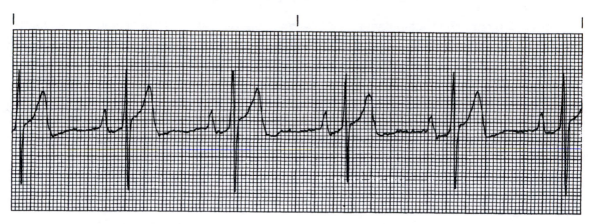

(Reprinted with permission from *Basic Arrhythmias, 3/E* by Gail Walraven,
Prentice Hall, Inc., Englewood Cliffs, NJ 07632.)

Regularity: _____
Rate: _____
P Waves: _____
PRI: _____
QRS: _____
Interp: _____

25. Fill in the information below for *normal sinus rhythm:*

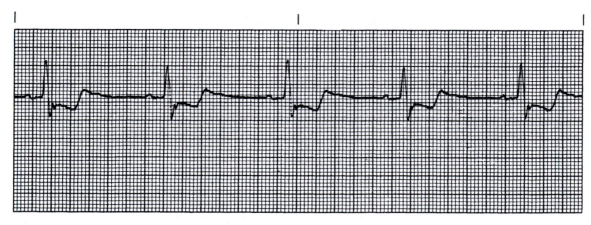

(Reprinted with permission from *Basic Arrhythmias, 3/E* by Gail Walraven,
Prentice Hall, Inc., Englewood Cliffs, NJ 07632.)

5.1   Regularity: _____
Rate: _____
P Waves: _____
PRI: _____
QRS: _____
Interp: _____

Clinical Disorders and Emergencies Affecting the Heart and Cardiovascular System

9

To provide the student with a basic understanding of the more frequently seen clinical disorders and emergencies affecting the heart and cardiovascular system.

COMPETENCY OBJECTIVES

Upon completion of this chapter, the student will be able to

1. Discuss and identify the clinical manifestations seen in heart disease.
2. Discuss and identify clinical disorders associated with the heart, including those which are congenital, inflammatory, and degenerative.
3. Describe what occurs during a myocardial infarction and identify an anterior, posterior, and diaphragmatic infarction.
4. Explain what occurs during heart failure.
5. Discuss and identify the clinical manifestations seen in disorders of the cardiovascular system.
6. Describe what occurs during ischemia and a cerebrovascular accident.
7. Explain what an aneurysm is.
8. Explain what hypertension is.

Cardiovascular disease, including those disorders affecting primarily the heart, is still considered one of the most widespread causes of death in the United States, accounting for more than 55 percent of all reported deaths in our population. The sad fact is that many of these deaths could have been avoided if early detection and treatment had been instituted early on in the illness.

There are nine classes of cardiovascular disease. These include congenital anomalies; rheumatic heart disease; inflammatory conditions, or diseases affecting the layers of the heart such as endocarditis, pericarditis, and myocarditis; arteriosclerosis; aneurysms; embolisms; neoplasms; peripheral vascular diseases; and ischemic heart diseases.

HEART DISORDERS: MANIFESTATIONS OF HEART DISEASE

In most cases of heart disease, the patient's symptoms will depend upon two manifestations: the nature of cardiopathy, and the resultant physiological disturbances in circulation. In addition, the majority of patients suffering from some type of cardiac disorder may also exhibit symptoms of discomfort involving breathing, pain, edema, or swelling of the tissues, palpitations, hemoptysis, or the coughing up of blood, fatigue, syncope, or fainting, and possibly some abdominal pain, discomfort, or other clinical manifestation of heart disease.

Dyspnea

The term *dyspnea* refers to an undue breathlessness and an awareness of discomfort associated with breathing. In cardiac patients, there is an increased effort in breathing due to a reduction of lung capacity resulting from pulmonary venous congestion.

Dyspnea due to heart disease is usually rapid and shallow, and the threshold, or tolerance for dyspnea, varies with the individual.

In cardiac patients we may see any one of four different types of dyspnea. One type, called *exertional dyspnea,* causes a breathlessness upon moderate exertion, usually relieved by rest, and primarily seen in congestive heart failure and chronic pulmonary disease. Another type, called *orthopnea,* creates a shortness of breath when lying down, which can only be relieved by promptly having the patient sit in an upright position. It is generally due to a stasis of blood accumulating in the lungs, indicating left ventricular failure or mitral disease.

A third type of dyspnea is *paroxysmal nocturnal dyspnea*. It comes on suddenly, usually at night while the patient is lying down, and is primarily due to left ventricular insufficiency, pulmonary edema, and mitral stenosis.

The last type of dyspnea seen in cardiac patients is called *Cheyne-Stokes respiration*. Here there is periodic breathing characterized by gradual increase in the depth of respirations, followed by a decrease in respiration, resulting in apnea. In other words, there are periods of increased respirations, called *hyperpnea*, with alternating periods of *apnea*, or no breathing. Cheyne-Stokes respiration is usually considered a serious sign and is primarily associated wtih left ventricular failure and cerebral vascular disease.

Chest Pain

Chest pain is generally considered one of the key signs of impending cardiac or cardiovascular problems. In the cardiac patient chest pain typically originates from ischemia, which is caused by stimulation of afferent nerve endings in the myocardium of the heart, resulting from oxygen deficiency in the cardiac muscle due to coronary artery disease.

Chest pain is predominantly characterized as excruciating or sharp precordial pain over the heart area and aggravated by deep breathing. Anxiety is generally considered a common cause of chest pain.

Edema

Edema is an abnormal accumulation of serous fluid in the connective tissues. It is generally caused by a build up of salt or sodium retention, and in the cardiac patient edema is most often seen in congestive heart failure.

Palpitation

Palpitation is defined as a rapid, forceful, or irregular heartbeat felt by the patient. Those patients suffering from palpitations usually complain of a pounding, jumping, stopping sensation in the chest. In cardiac disorders, palpitation is most often associated with enlargement of the heart and disturbances of rhythm.

Hemoptysis

Hemoptysis is the coughing up of blood. In cardiac patients, small quantities of dark, clotting blood usually indicate mitral stenosis, whereas a mixture of blood and pus may indicate pulmonary suppuration.

CLINICAL DISORDERS OF THE HEART

Congenital Anomalies

Congenital anomalies refer to those diseases and clinical disorders originating at birth. Two of the most common are called *patent ductus arteriosus* and *tetralogy of Fallot.*

Patent ductus arteriosus is considered a congenital lesion. In the fetus, the ductus arteriosus connects the pulmonary artery and the aorta, thus bypassing the lungs, which are not needed in utero. Shortly after birth the ductus should close to allow full utilization of the lungs. If the vessel remains open, blood laden with carbon dioxide will enter the aorta, thus reducing the oxygen supply to the tissues. This disorder can usually be corrected by surgery.

In tetralogy of Fallot, four lesions are present in the fetus's heart, which impair the supply of oxygen to the outlying tissues. These include a stenosis or narrowing at the pulmonary artery, consequent right ventricullar hypertrophy, interventricular septal defect, and a malpositioned aorta. Like patent ductus arteriosus, this disorder may be corrected surgically, early in the newborn's life.

Rheumatic Heart Disease

Rheumatic heart disease is a recurring febrile illness, more frequently seen in children than in adults. It affects the heart valves, usually damaging them, and the joints. Ultimately, stenosis develops and the valves must be replaced with artificial ones.

Inflammatory Conditions

Inflammation is generally seen in the three layers of the heart. In the endocardium it is known as *endocarditis;* in the pericardium, it is called *pericarditis;* and in the myocardium, it is referred to as *myocarditis.*

Endocarditis is an inflammation of the lining membrane of the heart. It is usually confined to the external lining of the valves, sometimes to the lining membrane of its chambers, and may be due to an invasion of microorganisms or an abnormal immunological reaction.

Pericarditis is an inflammation of the pericardium. In cardiac patients, it is usually associated with a myocardial infarction, neoplasm, or trauma to the heart, and it generally gives rise to symptoms such as moderate fever, precordial pain and tenderness, dyspnea, and palpitations.

Myocarditis refers to an inflammation of the myocardium, and can be associated with a number of conditions, including many types of infections, ingestion of poisons, such as carbon monoxide, and heat stroke and burns. It occurs commonly after rheumatic fever and diphtheria and rarely after viral infections.

ARTERIOSCLEROSIS

In arteriosclerosis, the interior walls of the blood vessels, especially the arteries, are subject to a buildup of hardened materials. Hence the term "hardening of the arteries."

There are two major types of arteriosclerotic diseases. The first, called *atherosclerosis,* is characterized by an accumulation of cholesterol built up within the arteries. In the second, called *arteriosclerosis,* coronary circulation is blocked, causing an ischemic heart disease to develop.

The major transient disorder of arteriosclerotic disease is called *angina pectoris.* Here the victim suffers occasional chest pain associated with temporary loss of blood supply to the myocardium. In more serious cases the arteriosclerotic plaque, or deposit, may cause a complete blockage of a cornary artery. This may lead to the death of the heart muscle tissue, or what is called a *myocardial infarction.*

MYOCARDIAL INFARCTION

A myocardial infarction, or what we commonly refer to as a "heart attack," is a result of a coronary artery becoming occluded. The severity of the infarction will depend greatly upon the state of the collateral circulation and the location of the occlusion. Unless blood flow is reestablished to the ischemic or dead tissue, more and more cells will succumb to the effects of anoxia, or lack of oxygen. In approximately 20 minutes, after the occlusion has occurred, the first necrotic (dead) cells begin to appear. Until this point, recovery would have been rapid with a reestablished blood flow, but necrosis is irreversible.

Ischemia of tissues surrounding the infarct causes a reversal of the T-wave. Because of the depolarization process is changed, owning to local ischemia the repolarization process is also altered.

Because of severe ischemia and lack of nutrients, the tissue immediately surrounding the center of the infarct is nonfunctional. It receives its blood supply from the collateral circulation. This is sufficient to keep it alive, but insufficient to maintain membrane integrity.

Nonfunctional or injured cardiac cells will begin to repolarize with the rest of the heart. However, a loss of membrane integrity makes it almost impossible for them to hold their charges. These charges, or ions, will then leak away from the cell. This exodus or exit of ions from the injured tissue is called a *current of injury.*

NECROSIS AND THE INFARCTION: THE EKG TRACING

Necrotic, or dead tissue, has no polarity. This area of the infarct therefore acts as a window through which the electrode "sees" a current moving away from the infarcted area. This abnormally directed QRS vector causes a Q-wave with a duration of more than 0.04 seconds in leads facing the infarcted area.

Myocardial necrosis, injury, and ischemia may be present at the same time, and the EKG manifestations of all three states may occur simultaneously. The positive electrode closest to the infarcted area will reflect the infarction most prominently.

Anterior Wall Infarction

The anterior wall is divided into four sections: anterobasal, anterolateral, anteroseptal, and apical. Infarctions may occur in all four areas.

The anterobasal, or hi-lateral infarct, is best seen on the EKG tracing in leads 1 and aV1 and is due primarily to an occlusion of a branch of the circumflex artery.

The anterolateral infarction is best seen on the tracing in the precordial leads overlying the infarct—that is, leads V4, V5, and V6. It is caused by an occlusion of the diagonal branch of the left anterior descending branch of the left coronary artery.

The anteroseptal or anterior infarct is best seen on the EKG tracing in leads V1, V2, and V3, and is due to an an occlusion of the left anterior descending branch of the left coronary artery.

Finally, the apical infarct is best seen on the tracing in leads 1 and aV1, and in the precordial leads V2, V3, and V4. It is caused by an occlusion of the left anterior descending branch of the left coronary artery.

Posterior Wall Infarction

A posterior wall infarction is caused by an occlusion of either the right coronary artery or a branch of the circumflex artery. In the EKG tracing, the precordial leads will show reciprocal changes caused by a loss of posterior forces. Therefore, instead of an abnormal Q-wave, there will be a tall, broad initial R. Instead of an S-T segment elevation due to an injury current traveling away from the electrode, there will be an S-T segment depression due to an injury current traveling toward the electrode. The T-wave will be upright rather than inverted. (See Figure 9–1.)

Diaphragmatic Infarction

The diaphragmatic infarction can best be seen on the EKG tracing in the limb leads II, III, and aVF. These are the leads in which the positive electrode "faces up" toward the infarcted area. It is caused by an occlusion of the right coronary artery.

Lateral Wall Infarction

A lateral wall infarction is caused by an occlusion of the circumflex artery or branch of the left anterior descending artery. The lateral wall of the heart faces up toward the left shoulder. Therefore, the positive electrodes that face this side of the heart will detect the infarction best. These leads are I, aVL, V5, and V6.

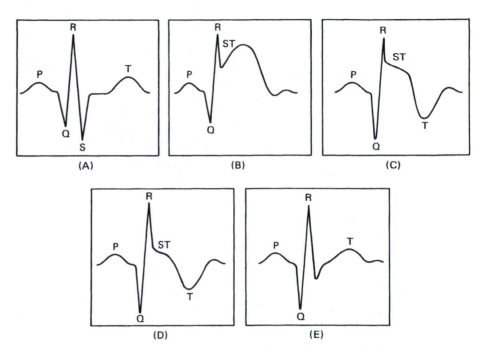

Figure 9-1 The myocardial infarction: (A) normal EKG tracing; (B) hours after infarction, S-T segment becomes elevated; (C) hours to days later, T-wave inverts, and Q-wave may become larger; (D) days to weeks later, S-T segment returns to near normal; (E) T-wave becomes upright again, but Q-wave may remain permanently large.

Stages of Recovery During an Infarction (See Figure 9-2.)

During the acute phases of an infarction, when there is a greater amount of nonfunctional and necrotic tissue present, S-T segment displacements and QRS changes are seen. As the nonfunctional tissue either dies or becomes functional again, the S-T segment displacements disappear and are replaced by inverted T-waves, an indication of secondary ischemia. The nonfunctional tissue in becoming functional will still be ischemic.

These processes take anywhere from several days to three weeks. As healing progresses, the Q-wave regresses. In most cases, it will persist permanently; however, at other times, the dead tissue becomes fibrosed and turns to scar tissue, and the area may be so small that it cannot even be detected on the EKG tracing.

HEART FAILURE

Heart failure is a general term meaning simply that the heart is no longer able to meet the body's demands. In either left heart failure or right heart failure, blood may pool in the body's tissues, causing ascites, or edema of the abdomen, and edema of the extremities. The lungs also become hypoxic, due to the lack of blood supply. Left heart failure causes pulmonary edema in the lungs and hypoxia of the systemic tissues.

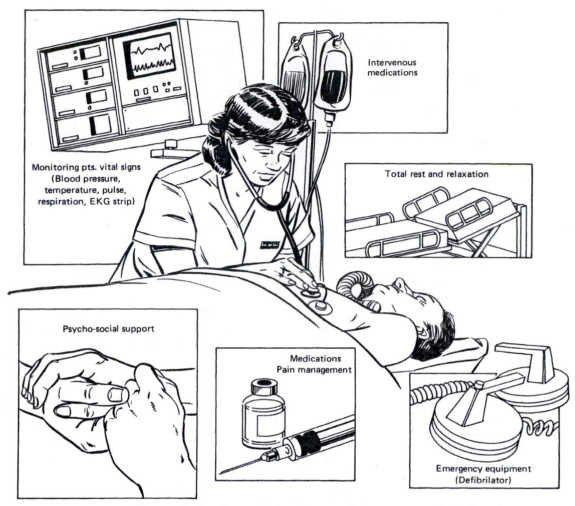

Figure 9–2   Stages of recovery after a myocardial infarction.

DISORDERS OF THE CARDIOVASCULAR SYSTEM

Although there are many disorders that may affect the entire cardiovascular system, few are generally seen without some involvement of the heart.

Manifestations of Vascular Disorders

As with cardiac disorders, diseases of the cardiovascular system are usually manifested by specific pathophysiologic symptoms. These include coldness, generally due to a deficient blood supply to a part even though the environment is warm; pallor or paleness, caused by a diminished blood supply, causing a lack of color in the individual afflicted; rubor, or redness, caused by impaired circulation; cyanosis, or blueness, generally an indication that less than a normal amount of oxygen is in the blood; and finally, pain, primarily due to an inadequate blood supply.

Varicose Veins

One type of cardiovascular disorder is known as *varicose veins.* In this condition there is an enlargement and twisting of the superficial veins. Varicose veins can occur in almost any part of the body, but they are most commonly observed in the lower extremity and in the esophagus.

Varicose veins are caused by incompetent venous valves that may be acquired or congenital. Their development is promoted and aggravated by pregnancy, obesity, and occupations requiring prolonged standing. Esophageal varices are caused by portal hypertension that accompanies cirrhosis of the liver. (See Figure 9–3.)

Ischemia and Cerebrovascular Accident (Stroke)

The two areas most frequently affected by arteriosclerosis are the cerebral and coronary vascular regions. Deposits in the intracranial vessels may

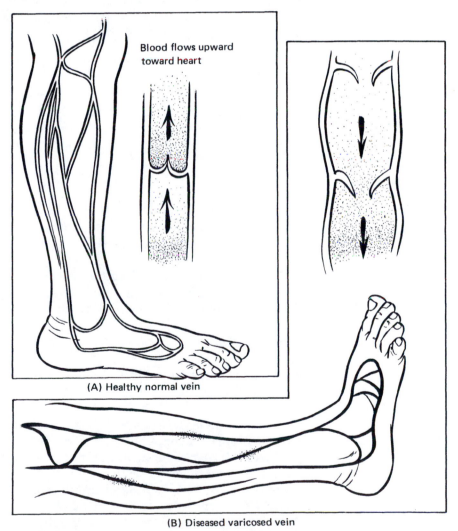

Blood flows upward toward heart

(A) Healthy normal vein

(B) Diseased varicosed vein

Figure 9–3 Comparison of healthy and diseased veins: (A) healthy normal vein; (B) diseased varicose vein.

TABLE 9–1
Classification of Diseases of the Cardiovascular System

Heart	Bacterial endocarditis, syphilis, pericarditis
Vascular system	Syphilitic vasculitis, arthritis, thrombophlebitis
Familial	Aneurysm
Traumatic	Incision, other wounds
Degenerative	Coronary heart disease, arteriosclerosis, myocardial infarction, angina atherosclerosis
Autoimmune	Rheumatic heart disease, endoccarditis, polymyositis
Neoplastic	Myxoma (heart muscle), hemangioma
Nutritional	Protein deficiency
Endocrine	Myxedema, acromegaly
Metabolic	Myopathy of heart muscle, hypertension
Psychiatric	Palpitation, hypertension
Congenital	Patent ductus arteriosus, atrial defects, tetralogy of Fallot, transposition of great vessels, coarctation, aneurysm

result, causing a condition known as *ischemia,* or lack of oxygen to the brain tissue.

A cerebrovascular accident, or "stroke," is a general term most commonly applied to cerebrovascular conditions that accompany either ischemic or hemorrhagic lesions. These conditions are usually secondary to atherosclerotic disease, hypertension, or a combination of both.

Aneurysms

Aneurysms are local dilations of blood vessels that bulge out from the vessel walls. They may be caused by an infectious process, such as syphilis, or as a result of conditions such as arteriosclerosis, congenital weaknesses, or trauma.

Aneurysms occur in several shapes and are described as saccular or dissecting. These lesions may eventually rupture and break open, and they can result in death from hemorrhage.

Hypertension

Hypertension, or high blood pressure, is a major class of cardiovascular disease. The three types of hypertension include essential, secondary, and renal.

While the exact cause of *essential* hypertension is not known, it is still considered a common health problem of the cardiovascular system. *Secondary* hypertension, on the other hand, is primarily associated with toxins, central nervous system (CNS) lesions, or endocrine disturbances; therefore, it is not seen as often as essential hypertension.

Renal hypertension is caused by excessive retention of sodium by the kidneys and is a problem frequently seen prior to onset of arteriosclerosis. Consequently, it is considered one of the most commonly treated disorders of the cardiovascular system.

REVIEW QUESTIONS

Directions: For the questions below, give the answers you believe are most correct:

1. Define the term *cardiovascular disease:*

2. What is the percentage of reported deaths occurring in the United States from cardiovascular disease?

3. List the five clinical manifestations of heart diease:

   (a) _____

   (b) _____

   (c) _____

   (d) _____

   (e) _____

4. Give at least one example of a congenital heart anomaly:

5. What occurs during endocarditis?

6. In heart patients, what is pericarditis usually associated with?

7. What does the expression "hardening of the arteries" refer to?

8. What is the main cause of a myocardial infarction?

9. What does "heart failure" represent?

10. List at least five clinical manifestations of cardiovascular disease:

    (a) _____

    (b) _____

    (c) _____

    (d) _____

    (e) _____

11. What occurs to the veins of a patient who is suffering from varicose veins?

12. What is an aneurysm?

13. What does the term *hypertension* mean?

14. Give an example of at least one degenerative heart disorder:

15. Give an example of at least one autoimmune disorder of the heart:

Understanding Vital Signs

10

TERMINAL OBJECTIVE

To provide the student with a basic understanding of vital signs, including temperature, pulse, respiration, and blood pressure, and the relationship of each to the body's proper function.

COMPETENCY OBJECTIVES

Upon completion of this chapter, the student will be able to

1. Describe the purpose of the temperature, pulse, respiration, and blood pressure, and the role each plays in the proper function of the body.
2. Describe the variations of temperature, pulse, respiration, and blood pressure.
3. Describe how to obtain a proper reading of the temperature, pulse, respiration, and blood pressure.

One of the best tools a physician has of evaluating a patient's physical condition is through the measurement of the vital or cardinal signs. These include temperature, pulse, respiration, and blood pressure. All are considered measurable, concrete indicators essential for life, and any deviation from what is considered the norm for each individual sign may provide the physician with a clear-cut symptom that one of the body systems is not functioning properly.

TEMPERATURE

Temperature is defined as the degree of body heat that is a direct result of the balance maintained between heat produced and heat lost by the body.

Many factors affect or influence body temperature. The time of day in which it is taken, for example, may affect the reading on the thermometer. Lowest body temperatures are usually registered in early morning, between the hours of 2:00 and 6:00, while the highest body temperature occurs in the evening hours, predominantly between the hours of 5:00 and 8:00.

The sex as well as the age of the patient also has a great deal to do with temperature. Women tend to increase their temperature during ovulation and pregnancy, and infants and children usually register a higher temperature than do adults.

Emotional status, degree of involvement in physical activity, and environmental changes are all factors tending to influence a patient's temperature. High temperatures usually occur during emotional excitement, such as when one is sad or angry, as well as during involvement in strenuous physical exercise. Emotions, as well as physical activity, will cause muscular contractions to occur in the body. On the other hand, changes in the weather, such as in cold climates, may tend to lower body temperature. This is due to the dilation of the blood vessels.

Methods of Measuring Temperature

Three acceptable methods exist for measuring body temperature. These include the most common method—taking the temperature orally—in which the thermometer is placed under the tongue; rectally, considered the most accurate method, in which the thermometer is placed in the rectum; and axillary, the least accurate of the three, in which the thermometer is placed under the axilla, or armpit. For children, the method of choice is rectal, and for children or adults who have difficulty holding an oral thermometer in place, the axillary method is considered most desirable.

Taking an Oral Temperature

As we have already stated, the most common method of taking a person's temperature is orally, or by mouth. Here the thermometer is held under the tongue and kept in place there for approximately 3 minutes. Normal readings for an oral temperature range from 97° to 99° Fahrenheit, with the average being 98.6° degrees Fahrenheit, or simply (F), or 37.5° Centigrade (or C). (See Figure 10–1.) When taking a patient's temperature by mouth, only an oral, "security," or "stubby" thermometer should be used. While all glass thermometers are calibrated in Fahrenheit or Centrigrade degrees and consist of two parts—the bulb and the stem—the oral thermometer has a long, slender bulb and therefore should never be inserted into the rectum. Security or stubby thermometers have a stubby round bulb that looks very much like a cross between an oral and rectal thermometer and therefore can be used to take either an oral or a rectal temperature.

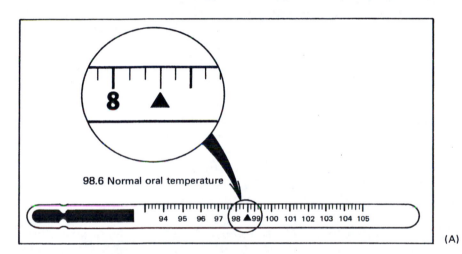

98.6 Normal oral temperature

(A)

(B)

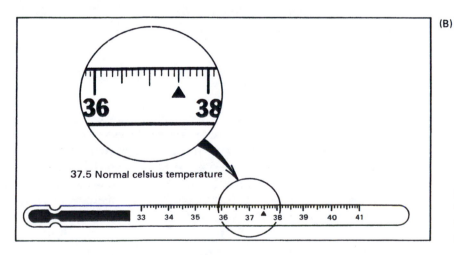

37.5 Normal celsius temperature

Figure 10–1 Reading the thermometer: (A) Fahrenheit thermometer; (B) Celsius thermometer.

Taking a Rectal Temperature

The taking of a rectal temperature is usually considered the method of choice for all infants and small children as well as for adults and older children who have difficulty holding an oral thermometer in place. In the rectal method, a rectal thermometer is used. It differs from the oral type in that it has a rounded short bulb that is better held by the rectal muscles. Both the security and stubby thermometers may also be used to take a rectal temperature. Whenever a rectal temperature is taken it is important to remember to leave the thermometer in place for approximately 5 minutes.

Taking an Axillary Temperature

The third and least accurate method of taking a temperature is by way of holding the thermometer in place between the inside of the upper arm and the axilla, or armpit. While it is acceptable to use either a security or stubby thermometer, this method is least desirable because of the length of time it takes to register a reading—that is, approximately 5 to 7 minutes, and because its accuracy of body temperature can vary and therefore is usually considered inaccurate.

Abnormal Body Temperature

As already noted, the average body temperature ranges from 97°F to 99°F, with the average being 98.6°. While the temperature reading for a rectal temperature usually averages 99.6°F and 97.6°F for an axillary temperature, anytime the body's temperature increases above 99.6°F there is a good indication that the patient may be suffering from some type of infection or dysfunctional medical condition.

Fever is referred to as *pyrexia,* and all fevers denote that the patient's oral temperature has risen above 98.6°F, or above normal. A low fever is one that ranges from 99° to 101°F (37.2° to 38.3°C). A moderate fever is defined as one ranging between 101° to 103°F (38.3° to 39.5°C). And a high fever is one ranging between 103° to 105°F (39.5° to 40.6°C).

THERMOMETERS

As already noted, three basic types of glass thermometers may be used to take an oral, rectal, or axillary temperature. However, other types of thermometers are acceptable for use in both the hospital and in private medical practices. These include disposable thermometers, which are made out of plastic or metal and usually contain indicator dots; the last dot to turn dark indicates the temperature reading; therefore, these thermometers are not considered to be highly accurate. There are also battery-operated electronic thermometers, which take a rapid and highly accurate temperature, and which come with disposable sheath covers and interchangeable color-coded probes for both oral and rectal use. In the battery-operated type, the temperature is registered on a dial, or a digital display. (See Figure 10–2.)

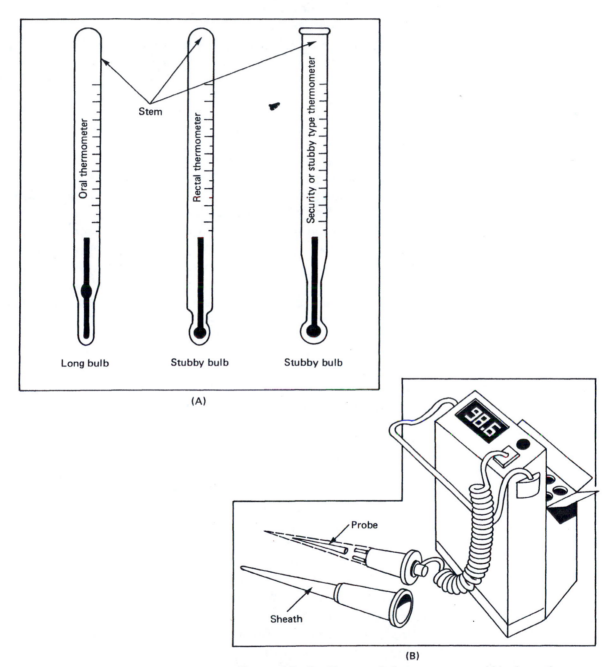

Figure 10–2 Types of thermometers: (A) glass thermometers; (B) battery-operated electronic thermometer.

PROCEDURES FOR TAKING AN ORAL TEMPERATURE

1. Gather the necessary equipment, including an oral thermometer (which should have been stored in a disinfectant solution such as 70% isopropyl alcohol) along with tissues or cotton balls, and Temp-a-Ways, if available.
2. Wash your hands.
3. Identify the patient and evaluate his or her condition. If the patient has had a hot or cold drink or has just finished eating or smoking, wait approximately 15 to 20 minutes before taking an oral temperature.
4. Ask yourself the following questions:
   (a) Is the patient a child six years of age or under?
   (b) Is the patient unable to breathe through his or her nose?
   (c) Is the patient uncooperative, delirious, or unconscious?
   If the answer to any of these questions is yes, do not take an oral temperature on the patient and check with the supervisor to see if another method should be used.
5. Position the patient sitting and explain the procedure.
6. Remove the oral thermometer from the solution and rinse with cold running water; wipe dry with tissues or cotton balls from the end of the stem to the bulb.
7. Check the mercury level of the thermometer. If the level is above 96°F, hold the thermometer firmly and shake downward with a snapping wrist movement.
8. If available, place the thermometer in a protective Temp-a-Way or plastic sheath and follow the manufacturer's directions.
9. Place the thermometer under the patient's tongue and instruct the patient to keep the mouth closed and breathe through the nose. Instruct the patient not to touch the thermometer with the teeth so as to avoid biting the thermometer.
10. Leave the thermometer in place for 3 minutes.
11. Remove thermometer and wipe once with a tissue or cotton ball from the end of the stem to the bulb; discard cotton ball or tissue and remove and discard Temp-a-Way if used.
12. Read thermometer by holding it horizontally and rotating it slowly until you see the column of mercury; read it exactly at the end of the mercury column.
13. Record the reading on the patient's chart where it is appropriate, making sure to record the method used.
14. Wash your hands.
15. Shake thermometer down again, so mercury falls below 96°F.
16. Wash the thermometer with soap and cold water and rinse with cold running water.
17. Place thermometer in disinfectant solution, such as 70% isopropyl alcohol.

18. If thermometer is not going to be reused within 24 hours, store it in a dry container.
19. Wash your hands after cleaning thermometer.

PROCEDURES FOR TAKING A RECTAL TEMPERATURE

1. Gather the necessary equipment, including a rectal thermometer, tissues, lubricant (such as K-Y Jelly), and Temp-a-Ways, if available.
2. Wash your hands.
3. Identify the patient and evaluate his or her condition as to whether or not a rectal temperature can be taken.
4. Explain the procedure.
5. If an adult, position the patient on the left side with the upper leg flexed at a 90° angle.
6. Remove the thermometer from the disinfectant solution, rinse, dry, and shake down the mercury level.
7. Use Temp-a-Ways, if available.
8. Lubricate the thermometer with the lubricant.
9. Separate the buttocks and expose the anus.
10. For an adult patient, gently insert the thermometer approximately 1 inch into the anal canal and instruct the patient to remain still.
11. Hold the thermometer in place for approximately 5 minutes.
12. Remove the thermometer and wipe from the stem to the bulb and read accurately.
13. Record the reading in the appropriate manner, making sure to record the method used.
14. Wash your hands.
15. Shake down the thermometer, wash, disinfect, and store it properly.
16. Wash your hands.

PROCEDURES FOR TAKING AN AXILLARY TEMPERATURE

1. Gather your equipment, including a stubby or security thermometer (stored in a disinfectant solution), tissues or cotton balls, and Temp-a-Ways, if available.
2. Wash your hands.
3. Identify the patient and evaluate his or her condition as to whether or not an axillary temperature can be taken.
4. Position patient sitting and explain the procedure.
5. Remove thermometer from solution, rinse, dry, and shake down mercury level.
6. Use Temp-aWays if available.

7. Place thermometer bulb in the hollow of the axillar, or armpit, and instruct patient to hold his or her arm across the chest or hold the opposite shoulder.
8. Leave thermometer in place for approximately 7 minutes.
9. Remove thermometer and wipe once with tissue or cotton ball from end of stem to the bulb; discard Temp-a-Way, cotton ball, or tissue.
10. Read thermometer.
11. Record reading in appropriate manner, making sure to put down method being used.
12. Wash your hands.
13. Shake down thermometer, wash, disinfect, and store.
14. Wash your hands.

MEASURING THE PULSE

Pulse is defined as the beat of the heart as felt through the walls of the arteries. It is the pulsation of the arteries produced by the wave of blood forced through them by the contractions of the heart.

A pulse is measured and recorded according to its individual characteristics. This includes the rate—that is, the number of pulsations or beats counted in a given minute; the rhythm, defined as the time interval between each pulse, usually described as regular, irregular, or skipping; and volume, or the strength of pulsations, described as full, strong, bounding, weak, or thready. A normal pulse is said to be regular and strong.

Pulse Sites

Since the pulse is the beat of the heart as felt through the walls of the arteries, it stands to reason that a pulse must be taken at a particular location or site—that is, at an artery.

The location of choice for taking a pulse on an average healthy person is at the radial artery located over the inner aspect of the wrist on the thumb side. This site is easily accessible and, therefore, is the most commonly used.

In addition to taking the pulse at the radial artery, pulse measurements may be taken at the brachial artery, located over the inner aspect at the bend of the elbow, or at the antecubital space, the temporal artery, located on the side of the forehead, at the temple; the carotid artery, located at the right and left sides of the anterior neck, and usually reserved for palpitation during CPR; the femoral artery, located at the anterior lower side of the hip bone in the groin region; the popliteal artery, located at the back of the knee; the dorsalis pedis artery, located on the upper surface of the foot between the ankle and the toes; and the apical site, located between the fifth and sixth ribs and approximately 2 to 3 inches to the left of the sternum. (See Figure 10–3.) When taking an apical

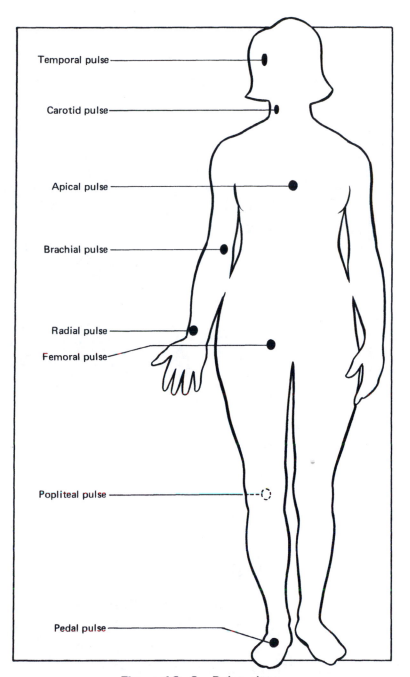

Temporal pulse

Carotid pulse

Apical pulse

Brachial pulse

Radial pulse

Femoral pulse

Popliteal pulse

Pedal pulse

Figure 10–3 Pulse sites.

pulse, a stethoscope must be used over the heart to measure the beats being produced. (See Figure 10–4.)

Pulse Rates and Variations

Pulse rates may vary and are influenced by many factors. These include the patient's age, sex, body size, emotional state, metabolism, and whether or not he or she is involved in exercise, taking drugs, is ill, or feeling pain.

For a normal, healthy adult, the average pulse ranges from 60 to 90 beats per minute, with 80 considered the norm. Children over seven

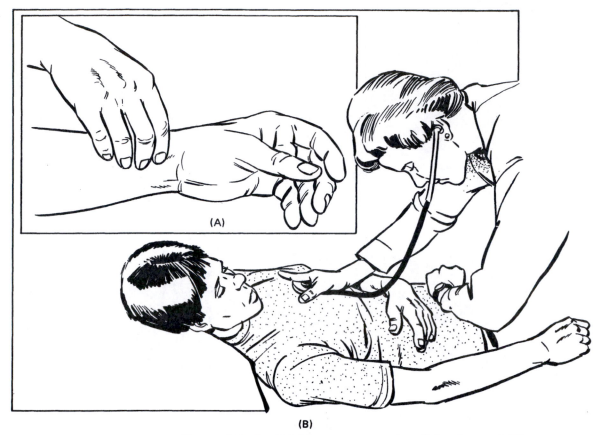

Figure 10–4   (A) Measurement of radial pulse and (B) auscultation of apical rate.

years of age range from 80 to 90 beats per minute, while children from the age of one to seven range from 80 to 120 beats per minute. Infants and newborns have the highest degree of pulsations, with a newborn ranging from 130 to 160 beats per minute and small infants ranging from 110 to 130 beats per minute.

PROCEDURES FOR OBTAINING A RADIAL PULSE RATE

1. Gather the necessary equipment, including a watch with a sweep second hand, and the patient's chart.
2. Wash your hands.
3. Identify the patient, explain the procedure, and evaluate his or her medical condition, making sure you do not take the reading immediately after the patient has become emotionally upset or after exertion, unless ordered by the physician.
4. Position the patient in a sitting or lying position, with the arm supported.
5. Hold the patient's wrist and place your first three fingers on his or her wristbone, over the radial artery. Apply light pressure so that

you can feel the pulsations. *Never* use your thumb to palpate the pulse.

6. Count the pulse for 60 seconds.
7. Note the rate, rhythm, and volume of the pulse.
8. Record the pulse rate, rhythm, and volume, and note the pulse site used, in the appropriate manner.
9. Wash your hands.

PROCEDURES FOR OBTAINING AN APICAL PULSE RATE

1. Gather the necessary equipment, including a stethoscope, watch with a sweep second hand, patient's chart, and an antiseptic wipe. (See Figure 10–5.)
2. Wash your hands.
3. Identify the patient, explain the procedure, and evaluate his or her medical condition; do not take the reading immediately after the patient has become emotionally upset or after any exertion, unless ordered by the physician.
4. Position the patient in a lying or sitting position.
5. Clean the earpieces of the stethoscope with an antiseptic solution.
6. Warm the diaphragm of the stethoscope with your hands to provide for patient comfort.
7. Place the earpieces of the stethoscope into your ears.
8. Place the diaphragm of the stethoscope over the apex of the heart, located in the fifth intercostal space, 2 to 3 inches to the left of the sternum.
9. Listen for the heartbeat and count the number of beats per minute.

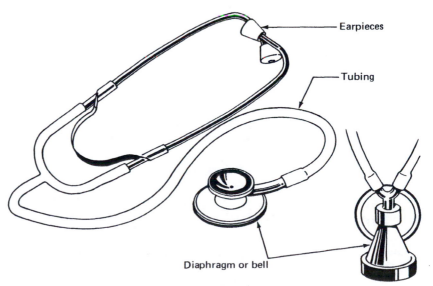

Earpieces

Tubing

Diaphragm or bell

Figure 10–5 Parts of the stethoscope.

10. Note the rhythm and volume.
11. Record the apical pulse rate, rhythm, and volume, indicating the site used, in the appropriate manner.
12. Clean the earpieces of the stethoscope.
13. Wash your hands.

MEASURING THE RESPIRATION

Respiration is defined as the act of breathing in oxygen and breathing out, or expiring, carbon dioxide. As with temperature and pulse, respiration is considered a vital sign, and any significant variation in its rate or rhythm is a clear indication that the body may not be functioning properly.

The process of respiration takes place in the respiratory control center, located in the medulla oblongata, or the lower portion of the brain stem. It is an act that occurs both automatically and through voluntary control. That is why an individual may hold his or her breath but eventually an involuntary breath must be taken in order to avoid passing out, or fainting.

Two types of respiration occur at the same time. The first, called *external respiration,* takes place as the exchange of respiratory gases between the alveoli of the lungs and the blood occurs. *Internal respiration* occurs with the exchange of respiratory gases between the body cells and the blood.

Respiration is characterized according to its rate, depth, and rhythm. *Rate* refers to the number of respirations per minute, and may be recorded as normal, rapid, or slow. *Depth* depends upon the amount of air being inhaled and exhaled and is recorded as shallow or deep. *Rhythm,* or the intervals of respiration, may be regular or irregular, in regard to the rate and depth.

Respiration Rates and Variations

Respiratory rates may vary. They are also influenced by a number of factors: the patient's emotional state, nervousness, increased muscular activity, the inducement of drugs into the blood stream, and any diseases of the lungs or circulatory system. In addition to these factors, certain climatic environments may also influence the respiratory rate. High altitudes, for example, tend to affect the rate and depth of the respirations, as do fever, sleep, and any dysfunction or injuries to the brain tissue.

PROCEDURES FOR OBTAINING A RESPIRATION RATE

1. Gather the necessary equipment, including a watch with a sweep second hand, and the patient's chart.
2. Wash your hands.
3. Identify the patient, explain the procedure, and evaluate the medical

condition. Do not take a respiration immediately after the patient has been emotionally upset or after any exertion, unless ordered by the physician.

4. Position the patient sitting or lying down.
5. Place three fingers on the patient's wrist, as if you were taking the pulse.
6. Count each breathing cycle (inhalation and exhalation) as one breath by watching the rise and fall of the chest or upper abdomen.
7. Count for one full minute.
8. Record the rate, depth, rhythm, and patient's position, in the appropriate manner.
9. Wash your hands.

BLOOD PRESSURE

The fourth and final vital sign most significant to the body's signaling of possible dysfunction is blood pressure. Defined as the pressure of the force of blood against the walls of the arteries, blood pressure is measured when the heart contracts and relaxes.

The process of blood pressure is actually divided into two separate functions. The first, called *systolic pressure,* is created when the force of blood is pushed against the artery walls when the ventricles of the heart are in a state of contraction. It is the upper number in a recorded blood pressure and is measured in millimeters of mercury (mmHg).

The second function, called *diastolic pressure,* occurs when the ventricles of the heart are in a state of relaxation. It is the lower number in the recorded blood pressure and is also measured in millimeters of mercury (mmHg).

Blood Pressure Variations

Blood pressure, like the other vital signs, may vary according to a number of factors, including age, sex, exercise, emotional state, drugs, increased weight or obesity, smoking, heart and renal diseases, and any condition of the blood vessels seen in old age. Additionally, blood pressure is usually higher when standing than when lying down and there is an increase of 3 to 4 mmHg higher in the right arm than in the left.

Normal blood pressure ranges anywhere from 110–140 systolic to 70–90 diastolic, or 110/70 to 140/90, with the average being 120/80 mmHg for a healthy adult. Because blood pressure increases with age, children usually run lower and older adults generally run higher.

Abnormal Blood Pressure Readings

As we have already stated, many factors can influence blood pressure. In certain instances, these factors become so out of sync with the body's cardiovascular system that the blood pressure either drops or increases to a point where the patient's life may be in danger.

The majority of abnormal blood pressure readings are divided into two major categories. Factors that cause the blood pressure to go below 110/70 mmHg result in a condition known as *hypotension,* while those factors that cause the blood pressure to rise above 140/90 mmHg are said to result in the disorder known as *hypertension.*

Although hypotension is more difficult to detect, for there are very few symptoms, except for general fatigue, associated with this condition, hypertension may be characterized by headaches, irritability, blurred vision, epistaxis, or nosebleed, nausea and vomiting, and vertigo, or dizziness.

Instruments Used for Measuring Blood Pressure

Two instruments are used to measure blood pressure. The first, called a *stethoscope,* consists of earpieces, tubing, and a diaphragm or bell. It is used to listen to beats of the heart as they are heard through the walls of the artery.

The second instrument used in the measurement of the blood pressure is the *sphygmomanometer.* It consists of four parts: a manometer, cuff, inflation bulb, and pressure control valve. The manometer is a gauge used to do the actual measurement of the blood pressure. There are two types most widely accepted. (See Figure 10–6.) The first, called a *mercury manometer,* uses a column of mercury to measure the blood pressure. It is most accurate and reliable because it does not have to be recalibrated, and can only be used when the column of mercury is in a vertical position.

The *aneroid manometer* may also be used for measuring blood pressure. It is a portable manometer that uses compressed air in order to measure the blood pressure. It differs from the mercury type in that it requires periodic calibrations.

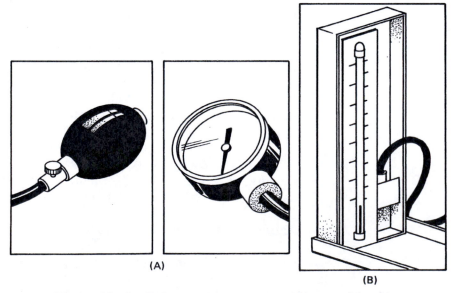

(A)

(B)

Figure 10–6 Sphygmomanometers: (A) aneroid sphygmomanometer; (B) mercury sphygmomanometer.

The cuff of the sphygmomanometer is made of an inflatable rubber bag covered with a nonstretch material, and which is wrapped around the patient's arm and secured with Velcro or clasps. Cuffs come in three sizes: pediatric, for children and for thin patients; adult, for normal size adults; and large, or obese, cuffs for adults with large arms or for use on a thigh.

The final two parts of the sphygmomanometer are the inflation bulb, which is used to pump air into a cuff through a rubber tube, and the pressure control valve, which is a thumbscrew valve located on the inflation bulb, used to allow air to escape as it is opened and closed.

PROCEDURES FOR MEASURING BLOOD PRESSURE
(See Figure 10-7)

1. Gather the necessary equipment, including a sphygmomanometer, stethoscope, 70% isopropyl alcohol, cotton balls or alcohol wipe, and the patient's chart.
2. Wash your hands.
3. Clean the earpieces and diaphragm or bell of the stethoscope with the alcohol.
4. Position the patient in a sitting position, with the arm supported; make sure patient is relaxed.
5. Expose the patient's arm by rolling up the sleeve approximately 5 inches above the elbow or remove the sleeve from the arm if necessary.
6. Place the deflated cuff evenly and snugly around the patient's arm with the lower edge approximately 1 to 2 inches above the antecubital space; center cuff over the brachial artery before securing with clasps or Velcro. If using a mercury manometer, place it on a level surface; if using an aneroid manometer, adjust it so the scale can be easily read.

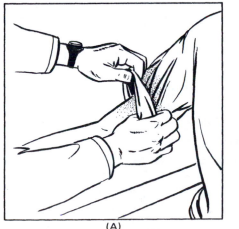
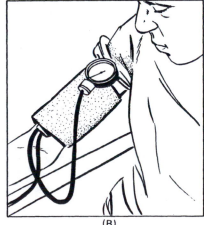

(A)   (B)

Figure 10-7 Measuring blood pressure: (A) Roll up the sleeve; (B) place cuff correctly on the arm;

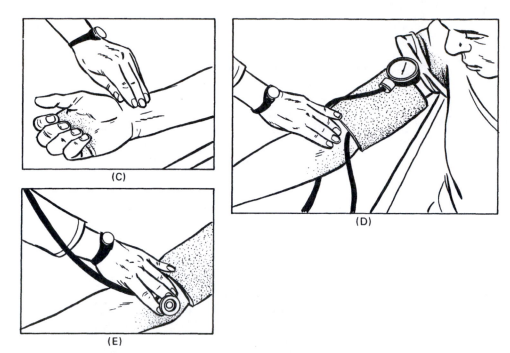

Figure 10–7 (cont.)   (C) palpate the radial artery; (D) find the brachial artery; (E) position stethoscope correctly.

7. Locate the brachial pulse in the antecubital space by palpating with your fingertips.
8. Place earpieces of stethoscope in your ears and place the diaphragm or bell gently but firmly over the brachial artery, making sure that the diaphragm or bell is not touching the cuff.
9. With the other hand, close the air valve on the bulb by gently turning the thumbscrew in a clockwise direction; pump air into the cuff until the level of the mercury is 10 to 20 mmHg above the palpated systolic pressure or about 180 mmHg.
10. Turn the thumbscrew counterclockwise to release the air at a slow rate, so that the pressure falls at approximately 2 to 3 mmHg per second.
11. Listen carefully for the first tapping sound; this represents the systolic pressure. Note this number on the scale of the aneroid manometer or the exact line on the mercury manometer.
12. Continue to deflate cuff while listening to the sounds. Read the scale again when the sound becomes dull or muffled; this represents the diastolic pressure.
13. Continue to deflate cuff at same speed until you no longer hear the sound.
14. Open the valve completely and rapidly deflate the cuff.
15. Remove the cuff from the patient's arm.
16. Record the results on the patient's chart, noting which arm was used, in the appropriate manner.
17. Wash your hands.

Follow-up Procedures

1. Take subsequent blood pressure readings using the same arm of the patient.
2. Take readings as quickly as possible; prolonged pressure affects the accuracy of the reading and is also very uncomfortable for the patient.
3. On all new patients, it is important to record the blood pressure in both arms. If a discrepancy occurs, use the arm with the higher reading in the future and record the discrepancy on the patient's chart.
4. Blood pressure should be taken routinely on all patients. Note any variations in blood pressure and report it to the physician, as required.
5. Periodically inspect sphygmomanometers for loss of mercury, or leaks in tubing, inflatable bag, or bulb.

REVIEW QUESTIONS

Directions: For the questions below, give the answers you believe are most
correct:

1. Define the term *temperature:*

2. When is body temperature the lowest? When is it the highest?

3. What are the three acceptable methods of taking the temperature? What
   is the least accurate method? What is the most accurate?

4. Define the term *pulse:*

5. Where is the location of choice for taking a pulse on an average healthy
   adult?

6. What is the name of the instrument used for both listening to the heart
   during a recording of an apical pulse and for taking the blood pressure?

7. Respiration is characterized according to its _____ ,
   _____ , and _____ .

8. Give at least one factor influencing respiration rates:

9. Define blood pressure:

10. When taking a blood pressure, the first reading made, when hearing the
    first of two consecutive sounds, is the _____ pressure;
    the second sound heard is the _____ pressure.

11. Generally, systolic blood pressure should remain below what level?

12. Generally, diastolic blood pressure should remain below what level?

13. You should never use your _____ to feel for the patient's pulse or blood pressure, since you may be feeling your own pulse.

14. What is considered the average "normal" blood pressure reading for a healthy adult?

15. What is the name of the instrument used to measure blood pressure?

Specialized Procedures Related to Electrocardiography

11

TERMINAL OBJECTIVE

To provide the student with a basic understanding of some of the more commonly performed specialized procedures related to the study of electrocardiography.

COMPETENCY OBJECTIVES

Upon completion of this chapter, the student will be able to

1. Discuss the importance of diagnostic evaluation for heart disease.
2. Describe the purpose and techniques involved in performing heart auscultation studies.
3. Describe the purpose of performing cardiographic studies.
4. Explain the purpose of an electrocardiogram.
5. Explain the purpose of ambulatory electrocardiographic monitoring.
6. Define the differences in performing a ballistocardiogram, phonocardiogram, and vectorcardiogram.
7. Explain what the purpose of echocardiography represents and briefly discuss how it is performed.
8. Describe the purpose of exercise stress testing.
9. Identify the most commonly performed radiological studies performed on the heart.
10. Discuss the purpose of angiocardiography and identify the types of angiocardiographic studies available.
11. Explain the purpose of performing a cardiac catheterization and identify the difference between a right-heart catheterization and a left-heart catheterization.

UNDERSTANDING THE NEED FOR DIAGNOSTIC EVALUATION FOR HEART DISEASE

In Chapter 9 we discussed some of the more dramatic disorders and emergencies affecting the human heart. Because many of these situations can manifest themselves into life-threatening circumstances, it is important that we spend some time discussing the need for their diagnostic evaluation.

Heart disease is still considered one of the major causes of death among our population. Therefore, it is important for the physician to diagnose and evaluate quickly any significant symptom related to heart disease that the patient presents. Then, and only then, is the doctor able to take the appropriate steps necessary in caring for the cardiac patient.

As a member of the cardiology team, the EKG technician is often involved in many of the studies and procedures available for diagnosing and evaluating the patient's heart. These diagnostic tools range from the recording of the basic 12-lead electrocardiogram, to many of the highly technological state-of-the-art cardiographic studies and procedures now available in many hospitals and medical centers throughout the country.

The majority of specialized cardiography procedures are classified into three major divisions: those involving some type of heart auscultation, or listening; those falling into the category of cardiographic studies; and those requiring some type of X-ray or radiological study.

HEART AUSCULTATION STUDIES

The process of heart auscultation requires that the technician be knowledgeable, have experience, and "tune in" a listening ear in order to hear each event occurring during the cardiac cycle. It is a systematic process in which the listener is required to use the stethoscope to "inch" from one area to another on the chest surface, always listening for any irregular sounds or beats the heart may be emitting.

The purpose of auscultation is to provide the physician with a means of measuring the rate and regularity or rhythm of the heart. It also determines whether or not the irregularity may be related to any respiratory movements. It may also be useful in evaluating the sequence in which an irregularity occurs.

In order to perform the heart auscultation properly, the listener is also required to assess the patient's venous pulse. This is done by having the examiner carefully "feel" for the pulsation in both the right carotid artery and in the radial artery. Once the pulsations have been felt, the examiner then feels for any precordial movement as he or she listens to the heart sounds.

CARDIOGRAPHIC STUDIES

The majority of studies and procedures used in the diagnostic evaluation of heart disease fall primarily into the cardiographic category. These are tests, usually performed with the help of noninvasive equipment, that provide the physician with an opportunity to "see" or "listen" to what the diseased heart may be doing. They range from the standard 12-lead electrocardiogram to high-tech ultrasonic listening devices that produce an echocardiogram. And their usefulness depends mainly on what the physician is looking for in the diseased heart.

The Electrocardiogram

As we have already discussed, the electrocardiogram (EKG) represents a visualization of the electrical activity of the heart as it is reflected by changes in the electrical potential on the skin's surface. It is obtained by placing leads on various body parts and then recording the electrical impulses as "tracings" on a strip of paper or on the screen of an oscilloscope.

The EKG is most useful in the evaluation of conditions that interfere with normal electrophysiological function of the heart, as well as in the evaluation and diagnosis of disturbances involving rhythm, disorders of cardiac muscle, enlargement of the chambers of the heart, and any potential electrolyte disturbances.

The electrocardiogram is almost always performed by the EKG technician, who is also responsible for gathering and writing any data pertinent to the patient. This includes the age, blood pressure, any symptoms that might be present, and any medications, especially those affecting the heart such as digitalis or any diuretics, prior to recording the electrocardiogram. (See Figure 11–1.)

Ambulatory Electrocardiographic Monitoring

This procedure requires that the patient wear a miniaturized tape-recording device that uses a single- or double-lead system attached to a belt or which is worn as a shoulder device.

Also known as a Holter monitor, various systems of this method of scanning the heart are available for recording the patient's electrocardiographic readings continuously for up to 24 hours while he or she goes about daily activities.

This procedure is most useful in determining the effects of arrhythmias, in assessing the patient's response to therapy, and in the evaluation of patients after they have sustained a myocardial infarction.

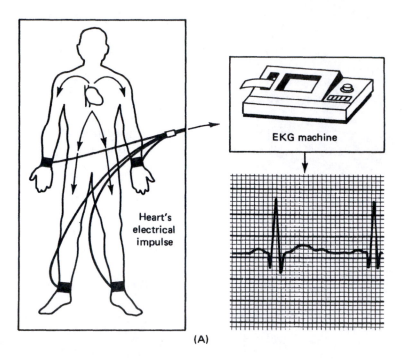

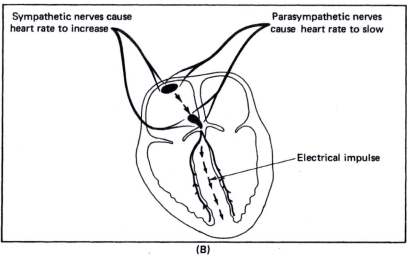

Figure 11–1 (A) Transmission of heart's impulse during the electrocardiogram; (B) heart physiology during the electrocardiogram.

Ballistocardiogram

Although performed infrequently, this procedure is most useful when a physician requires a graphic representation of the recording of the movement of the body generated with each heartbeat. By doing so, it provides information on the strength and coordination of cardiac contractions.

Phonocardiogram

The purpose of a phonocardiogram is to provide the physician with a graphic recording of the occurrence, timing, and duration of the sounds in the cardiac cycle. While it is a process that may be completed simultaneously with the recording of the electrocardiogram, it is also considered a highly technical procedure involving detection, through a highly sensitive microphone, of sonic vibrations from the heart, which are then converted into electrical energy and fed into a galvanometer, where they can be recorded onto paper.

This procedure is most useful when the physician believes there is evidence of heart murmurs or unusual heart sounds, such as gallops, that otherwise may be difficult to discern by the human ear.

Vectorcardiography

This procedure represents a method of recording the magnitude and the electrical action of the heart in the form of a vector loop display on a cathode ray oscilloscope. Performing this test provides the physician with an analysis of the configuration of these loops and therefore permits certain assessments to be made about the state of health or diseased condition of the myocardium of the heart. At any particular moment the electrical activity of the heart can be represented as an electrical vector with a specific direction and magnitude. This makes this test most useful for the physician when diagnosis of electrical activity of the atrium or ventricles is necessary.

Echocardiography

Echocardiography is considered one of the most useful tools necessary in diagnosing any demonstration of valvular or other structural deformities present in the heart. It is also helpful in detecting the presence of pericardial effusion and in assisting the physician in the diagnosis of a cardiac tumor, heart enlargement, or in any prosthetic valve function or dysfunction.

The process of echocardiography involves obtaining a recording of the position and motion of the heart walls or internal structures of the heart and neighboring tissue by the echo emanating from beams of ultrasonic waves directed through the chest wall. It is based upon the technique of depth-sounding—that is, it utilizes ultrasound in order to delineate the anatomical structures by recording on a graph the echoes from the heart structures.

Also referred to as *ultrasound cardiography,* echocardiography is responsible for creating a record of high-frequency sound vibrations that have been sent into the heart through the chest wall. The cardiac structures return the echoes derived from the ultrasound. It accomplishes this through the motions of the echoes being traced on an oscilloscope and then recorded onto film. (See Figure 11–2.)

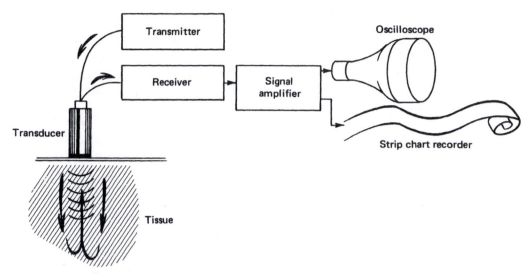

Figure 11-2 Schematic drawing of the echograph machine.

EXERCISE STRESS TESTING

Exercise stress testing is a procedure completed by the patient through the use of a treadmill or bicyclelike device and is used as a means of evaluating the patient's circulatory response to stress. As the patient is performing the exercise, the stress test evaluates the patient's capacity for physical performance while also evaluating any electrophysiological abnormalities that may indicate myocardial ischemia.

This procedure is also useful in evaluating and diagnosing any occult heart conditions that may be present. It may only be performed under the direct supervision of the physician and is completed while the patient is exercising, by increasing his or her walking speed and the incline of the treadmill, or by increasing the load against which pedaling occurs.

RADIOLOGICAL STUDIES OF THE HEART

Studies and procedures falling into this category involve two methods of X-raying or visualizing the heart's performance and capacity to function properly. The first method involves the actual visualization of the heart through either X-rays or fluoroscopy, whereas the second method entails more precise testing, usually through the employment of secondary testing, as in the process of introducing intravenous dyes into the bloodstream for more detailed visualization of the heart's structure. This latter method of testing involves the use of *angiocardiography.*

Chest X-Ray and the Heart

The most basic of all radiological (or roentgenological) studies of the heart involve the taking of a chest X-ray. Its purpose is to provide the physician with a tool for evaluating and diagnosing conditions of the heart related to its size, contour, and position, as well as to provide additional information that may demonstrate early interstitial pulmonary edema.

Planigraphy and the Heart

This radiological study is primarily ordered when the physician chooses to look at a specific body section. In relation to the heart, planigraphy allows the examiner to identify the cardiac contour that may have been obscured by a regular chest X-ray. It is also useful in identifying and localizing intracardiac and vascular calcification.

Fluoroscopy and the Heart

The procedure known as *fluoroscopy* is a useful tool for the physician in assessing unusual cardiac contours and valvular pulsations. The procedure is accomplished through the recognition of the contours and pulsations on a luminescent X-ray screen. Its usefulness is also important in verifying the position of intravenous pacemaking electrodes and for guidance of the catheter during cardiac catheterization.

UNDERSTANDING ANGIOCARDIOGRAPHY

The use and implementation of angiocardiography as a diagnostic tool for evaluating a diseased heart has afforded physicians a method by which to X-ray both the vascular system of the heart and the cardiovascular system. Angiocardiography involves the injection of a contrast medium into the vascular system, which is used as a means of outlining the heart and blood vessels, while accompanied by serial radiographs, or photographs, being taken through the use of high-speed motion picture film. Thus, angiocardiography provides the physician with information regarding any structural abnormalities, such as occlusions, defects, fistulas, or abnormal valve function, that may affect the heart.

Types of Angiocardiography

There are three basic types of angiocardiography procedures performed on most cardiac patients. The first, called *selective angiocardiography,* is performed by injecting a contrast medium through a catheter directly into one of the coronary arteries, or greater vessels. The angiocardiogram is then recorded by means of a rapid film changer or motion picture camera.

The second type of angiocardiography performed is called *aortography.* It is useful in the diagnosis of disease or dysfunction of the lumen of the aorta and the major arteries arising from it. The third procedure, called *thoracic* aortography, involves the introduction of a contrast medium, which outlines the aortic arch and its great vessels. These can then be studied by means of rapid serial radiographs, or roentgenograms.

Coronary Arteriography

Coronary arteriography is defined as a technique in which a radiopaque catheter is introduced into the right brachial artery, via open arteriotomy (or femoral artery via percutaneous puncture), passed into the ascending aorta, and then manipulated into the appropriate coronary artery, under fluoroscopic control.

This procedure is most useful as a diagnostic tool in evaluating the patient for coronary artery surgery or myocardial revascularization, and after surgery in order to evaluate graft patency. It can also be useful in studying any suspected congenital anomalies of the coronary arteries. (See Figure 11–3.)

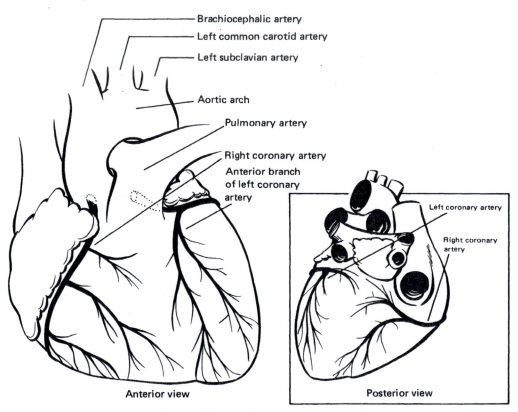

Figure 11–3 The coronary arteries.

CARDIAC CATHETERIZATION

The process of performing a cardiac catheterization is almost always used by the physician in helping to determine either the extent of injury to a diseased heart or as a preliminary test prior to the patient undergoing heart surgery. It involves the passage of a catheter into the heart and blood vessels and is used as a diagnostic tool in measuring oxygen concentration, saturation, and pressure in the various heart chambers. It is also useful in detecting any shunts, in providing blood samples for analysis, and in determining cardiac output and pulmonary blood flow. The use of cardiac catheterization is almost always combined with angiocardiography for visualization of the coronary arteries.

Types of Cardiac Catheterization

There are two types of cardiac catheterization. The first, called a *right-heart catheterization*, is performed by passing a radiopaque catheter from an antecubital or femoral vein into the right atrium, right ventricle, and pulmonary vasculature, under direct visualization with a fluoroscope. This procedure can be used to measure the pressures of both the right atrium and the right ventricle. During this procedure, the catheter is introduced into the pulmonary artery and as far as possible beyond that point. Capillary samples and capillary wedges can then be recorded.

In the second type of cardiac catheterization, called a *left-heart catheterization*, the procedure is accomplished using four sites: a precutaneous needle puncture of the left atrium, a precutaneous needle puncture of the left ventricle, a transeptal puncture, and a retrograde puncture of the left ventricle. By using all four sites, the physician is given an exact picture of the flow and pressure measurements of the left heart. It also provides a useful method of evaluating the status of the mitral and aortic valves and coronary arteries.

Because cardiac catheterization does involve the introduction of a foreign object directly into the heart's structure, there is always a possibility of complications arising from this procedure. Some of these complications include arrhythmias, such as ventricular fibrillation, pericardial tamponade, myocardial infarctions, and pulmonary edema. Thrombophlebitis, or inflammation of the vein being used for the catheterization, may also occur, as well as allergic reactions to the contrast dye.

While many of the pre- and postcatheterization considerations necessary for caring for the patient are almost always the responsibility of the nursing care team, it is important that the EKG technician who may be involved in this procedure be aware of some of the prior and post-patient care implications involved in this test. These include being knowledgeable in the approach being used; making sure that all food and fluids have been withheld from the patient for at least 6 hours prior to the procedure; ascertaining a history of any previous allergies, particularly if they are related to a contrast medium; removing the patient's dentures prior to the exam; and finally, making sure that the patient has been properly premedicated, as directed by the physician, prior to the procedure.

Once the procedure is complete, the patient is monitored electro-cardiographically and the vital signs recorded at least every 15 minutes until they are stable. Peripheral pulses, temperature, and color of the affected extremity are also noted, as well as any complaints by the patient of pain, numbness, or tingling sensations, all of which may be indicative of possible arterial insufficiency.

REVIEW QUESTIONS

Directions: For the questions below, give the answers you believe are most correct:

1. _____ _____ is still considered one of the major causes of death among our population.

2. Identify the three major classifications of specialized cardiography procedures:

   (a) _____

   (b) _____

   (c) _____

3. The purpose of _____ is to provide the physician with a means of measuring the rate and regularity of the heart.

4. In _____ _____ _____ _____ , the patient wears a miniaturized tape-recording device attached to his or her clothing, for the purpose of recording electrocardiographic readings continuously for up to 24 hours.

5. A _____ is a representation of the recording of the movement of the body generated with each heart movement.

6. The physician may order a _____ if he or she believes there is evidence of a heart murmur.

7. _____ is a method used for recording the magnitude and electrical action of the heart.

8. The purpose of _____ is to create a record of high-frequency sound vibrations that have been sent into the heart through the chest wall.

9. The most basic of all radiological (roentgenological) studies of the heart is the _____ _____ .

10. The use of _____ provides the physician with information regarding any structural abnormalities such as occlusions, defects, fistulas, or abnormal valve function affecting the heart.

11. The process of _____ _____ is almost always used as a preliminary test prior to the patient undergoing heart surgery.

Pharmacology
and Electrocardiography

12

TERMINAL OBJECTIVE

To provide the student with a basic understanding of some of the more commonly used drugs and medications implemented in the treatment of cardiac disorders.

COMPETENCY OBJECTIVES

Upon completion of this chapter, the student will be able to

1. Correctly spell and define terminology related to pharmacology and its use in performing electrocardiography.
2. Explain the use, purpose, function, and effects of cardiac glycosides.
3. Explain the use, purpose, function, and effects of antiarrhythmic drugs.
4. Discuss the difference between Class I, Class II, Class III, and Class IV antiarrhythmic drugs.
5. Explain the use, purpose, function, and effects of antianginal agents.
6. Discuss the differences between nitrites and nitrates; between beta blockers and calcium antagonists.
7. Explain the use, purpose, function, and effects of diuretics.

DRUGS AND THE TREATMENT OF CARDIAC CONDITIONS

The use of certain drugs in the treatment of specific cardiac medical conditions is practiced by the majority of physicians in the care of their patients. These medications may have a number of effects on the diseased heart, including increasing or decreasing the strength or action of the heart, increasing the cardiac output, and keeping the heart beating in an even, non-life-threatening way. The EKG technician has a responsibility both to know and understand the purpose and effects of these drugs, for their use may have a direct result on the electrocardiogram.

UNDERSTANDING CARDIAC GLYCOSIDES

Cardiac glycosides are primarily given to patients who suffer from the disease known as congestive heart failure, or CHF. When this disease occurs, the body tries to reverse the effects of heart failure by stimulating compensatory reflexes involving the sympathetic nervous system. Sympathetic reflexes release norepinephrine and epinephrine, which in turn cause vasoconstriction, or a tightening of the blood vessels, and an increased heart rate and force of contraction in the heart. These effects are an attempt to increase the blood flow and thereby relieve the congestion.

Patients who suffer from CHF use drug therapy involving the use of digitalis or what we refer to as *cardiac glycosides*, whose action includes the force of myocardial contraction. These almost always require the use of *diuretics*, which help to eliminate excess sodium and water,

TABLE 12-1
Commonly Used Cardiac Glycosides

Drug name	Route	Oral dose for maintenance (mg)	Peak effect (hours)
Acetyldigitoxin	P.O.	0.1–0.2	8–10
Deslanoside	I.M., I.V.	—	2–4
Digitalis	P.O., I.V.	50–200	8–24
Digitoxin	P.O., I.V.	0.05–0.2	8–12
Digoxin	P.O., I.V.	0.125–0.5	6
Gitalin	P.O.	0.25–1.25	8–10
Quabain	I.V.	—	—

and vasodilator drugs, which indirectly increase the amount of blood pumped by the heart, or what we refer to as *cardiac output*.

The cardiac glycosides are a group of compounds obtained from the plant leaves of *Digitalis purpurea* and *Digitalis ianata*. These compounds, known as glycosides, are similar in chemical and pharmacological properties. Digitalis, the oldest preparation made from the dried and powdered leaf of *Digitalis purpurea*, is a combination of several individual glycosides mixed in one preparation. Most of the other preparations contain only one glycoside. (See Table 12–1.)

UNDERSTANDING THE PHARMACOLOGICAL EFFECTS OF GLYCOSIDES

The unique pharmacological effect of the cardiac glycosides is to increase the force of myocardial contraction that has occurred during congestive heart failure, without causing an increase in the amount of oxygen consumed. A second important effect of these drugs is that the heart rate and AV conduction are decreased. This effect is caused by the action of the glycosides in stimulating the vagus nerve. In addition, the glycosides also act as a direct depressant on the AV node.

Glycosides also produce several characteristic changes in the patient's electrocardiogram. At therapeutic doses, there is a depression of the S-T segment as well as changes in the T-wave. Additionally, there is a lengthening of the P-R interval, which reflects slower conduction through the AV node. At higher doses, the decreased conduction through the AV node can lead to various degrees of heart block.

Cardiac glycosides increase the force of myocardial contraction by increasing the entry of calcium inside the cardiac muscle cells. The efficiency of muscle contraction depends upon the calcium that initiates the formation of actinomysin, resulting in myocardial contraction.

The administration of glycosides normally follows a sequence, known as "digitalization and maintenance." During the digitalization phase, glycosides are administered either orally or intravenously, at doses and intervals that rapidly produce an effective blood level. Additional maintenance doses are lower, usually one-fourth of the digitalizing dose, and are then adjusted in order to maintain a therapeutic level of glycoside in the blood. An accumulation of the drug in the body can result in toxic effects; therefore, it is important that routine determinations of blood levels containing the glycosides be done so as to avoid cumulative effects of these drugs.

Digoxin and digitoxin are two of the most widely used glycosides. Both can be administered either orally or intravenously depending on the urgency of the situation. Food may delay absorption of the glycosides but usually does not interfere with the extent of absorption. Digoxin is not bound significantly to plasma proteins and is therefore excreted mostly unmetabolized by the urinary tract.

The major adverse effects of the glycosides are caused by overdose. Mild symptoms include nausea, vomiting, headache, visual disturbances, and rashes; dose reduction is usually sufficient to relieve these symptoms.

In some cases the cardiac glyosides may produce adverse effects considered to be life-threatening. Patients taking these drugs should always be made aware of the common side effects, such as nausea, vomiting, diarrhea, loss of appetite, visual disturbances, headache, or increased feelings of tiredness, all of which may be an indication of an impending drug accumulation. Thus, it is extremely important that patients receiving glycosides be given proper instruction as to the importance of notifying their physician if any of these symptoms start to occur. Profuse vomiting and diarrhea, for example, are two symptoms, which left untreated, could lead to an alteration of the electrolyte levels in the blood, which can ultimately contribute to digitalis toxicity. This alteration is especially likely in patients who are also taking thiazide or any other organic acid diuretic.

ANTIARRHYTHMIC DRUGS

Disorders in the cardiac rhythm, referred to as *arrhythmias,* are the most commonly occurring pathophysiological conditions. Arrhythmias may develop in a diseased heart, as a result of congestive heart failure, coronary artery disease, myocardial infarction, or as a consequence of chronic drug therapy. The symptoms of a rhythm disorder may range from mild palpitations to cardiac arrest, and the severity of these symptoms usually determines the overall effect on cardiac function and blood pressure.

The clinical management of an abnormal cardiac rhythm involves a group of pharmacological agents responsible for converting the existing arrhythmias to a normal rhythm, thereby preventing future arrhythmias. (See Table 12–2).

Class I Antiarrhythmic Drugs

Class I antiarrhythmic drugs have one very common feature: They also possess an anesthetic property. Like local anesthetics, the Class I drugs interfere with the movement of sodium ions during excitation and depolarization of the cardiac membranes. Consequently, the excitability of the heart is reduced, particularly any areas of the heart that are hyperexcitable and arrhythmogenic—that is, giving rise to an arrhythmia. In addition, Class I drugs slow conduction velocity, prolong the refractory period, and decrease automaticity of the heart. All of these actions may contribute to the antiarrhythmic effect.

The five drugs most frequently referred to as Class I antiarrhythmics include quinidine, procainamide, disopyramide or Norpace (trade name), lidocaine, and phenytoin.

Quinidine is considered a general cardiac depressant—that is, it depresses the myocardial and conduction systems of the heart. The overall effect of quinidine is to slow the heart rate; however, quinidine initially exerts an anticholingeric effect on the SA node, which may result in tachycardia, or an abnormally fast heartbeat, eventually worsening an existing arrhythmia being treated.

TABLE 12-2
Antiarrhythmic Drug Interactions

Antiarrhythmic agent	Interacts with	Interaction
Phenytocin	Oral antidiabetics Tolbutamide	Hyperglycemia; ataxia; polydipsia; polyuria
	Disulfiram	Increases blood phenytoin level
	Alcohol	Decreases blood phenytoin level
Propranolol	Insulin	Hypoglycemia
Quinidine	Antibiotics Kanamycin Neomycin Streptomycin	Paralysis of respiratory muscles
	Anticoagulants	Increases bleeding
	Antiinflammatory agents	Increased quinidine toxicity
	Anticholinergics	Tachycardia
	Barbituates	Increased quinidine toxicity
	Cardiac glycosides Digoxin	Increased digitalis toxicity
	Diuretics Acetazolamide Hydrochlorothiazide	Increased quinidine toxicity
	Neuromuscular blockers	Paralysis of respiratory muscles
	Potassium salts	Increased quinidine toxicity
	Reserpine	Excessive bradycardia

Procainamide, another frequently used Class I antiarrhythmic drug, produces the same pharmacological actions as quinidine. Although this drug produces very few side effects in therapeutic doses, the common side effects are nausea, vomiting, anorexia, and skin rashes. Procainamide is also capable of producing changes in the electrocardiogram, which are similar to quinidine, such as the intervals widening in the P-R, QRS, and T intervals. Usually these widenings occur along with the appearance of premature beats.

Disopyramide, or Norpace, produces effects similar to those of quinidine and procainamide. It usually causes a decrease in the excitability and prolongation of the refractory period, and is most commonly used in the treatment of both atrial and ventricular arrhythmias. The drug is a general cardiac depressant, and at higher doses, or with the development of toxicity, may produce quinidinelike depression of the heart.

The fourth Class I antiarrhythmic drug used most frequently is a synthetic drug called lidocaine. Although the drug is used primarily as a local anesthetic agent, it is also widely promoted for use during ventricular arrhythmias, especially those resulting from a myocardial infarction or during surgery. The main effect of this drug is in the prevention of ventricular arrhythmias. The major disadvantage, however, is that it must always be administered intravenously.

The last Class I antiarrhythmic drug, phenytoin, finds its greatest use as an antiepileptic drug; however, it may also be recommended in the treatment of ventricular arrhythmias, especially those induced by digitalis, such as in the case of an AV block. The most common side effects of phenytoin include blurred vision, vertigo, and nystagmus, or involuntary movement of the eyes, accompanied by dizziness. Administration of the drug in large doses may also result in an elevated blood glucose level.

Class II Antiarrhythmic Drugs

Class II antiarrhythmic drugs are referred to as *beta-adrenergic blockers*, responsible for increasing the heart rate, excitability, conduction velocity, and automaticity, particularly those of ventricular muscle. In addition, they also shorten the refractory period. The use of these drugs, although classified as antiarrhythmic, may also lead to the increased development of arrhythmias.

The only beta blocker used as an antiarrhythmic drug is propranolol. It produces an effect similar to that of quinidine in that it depresses the cardiac membranes at higher doses. Both supraventricular and ventricular arrhythmias can be treated with propranolol. In addition to its own use as a single anitarrhythmic drug, propranolol may also be used in conjunction with Class I antiarrhythmics when control is not achieved with one drug alone.

Class III Antiarrhythmic Drugs

The drugs grouped together as Class III antiarrhythmic drugs include only one FDA-approved drug, called bretylium, or Bretylol (trade name). This drug is an adrenergic neuronal blocker, which decreases the release of norepinephrine from adrenergic nerve endings. In addition, bretylium also prolongs the refractory period of the ventricles. This action is useful in the treatment of resistant ventricular tachycardia and ventricular fibrillation.

Class IV Antiarrhythmic Drugs

Class IV antiarrhythmic drugs are the newest antiarrhythmic drugs and are referred to as *calcium antagonists*. The purpose of these drugs is to decrease the entry of calcium inside the cells that have electrophysiological properties—that is, those cells with excitable membranes which develop action potentials. Such cells include those of the heart and blood vessels.

One of the calcium antagonists, verapamil, is now used for its antiarrhythmic actions. Its major effect is on the pacemaker cells of the heart. It decreases the SA node activity, resulting in a slight decrease in the heart rate. More importantly, verapamil decreases the AV node conduction, making it a very useful drug in the treatment of various types of AV nodal arrhythmias. (See Table 12–3.)

TABLE 12–3
Antiarrhythmic Drugs and Their Uses

Drug name	Arrhythmias treated	Average dose
Quinidine	Supraventricular tachy-arrhythmias, ventricular arrhythmias	200–400 mg BID, TID P.O.
Procainamide	Supraventricular tachy-arrhythmias, ventricular arrhythmias	250–500 mg QID P.O.
Disopyramide	Ventricular arrhythmias	100–200 mg TID, QID P.O.
Lidocaine	Ventricular arrhythmias	1–2 mg/kg bolus I.V. 1–4 mg/min infusion
Propranolol	Supraventricular and ventricular tachy-arrhythmias	40–80 mg TID, QID P.O. 1.0–3.0 mg twice at 2-min intervals if necessary in any 4-hour period
Verapamil	Supraventricular tachy-arrhythmias	80–120 mg TID, QID P.O.; 5–10 mg I.V.

UNDERSTANDING ANTIANGINAL AGENTS (VASODILATORS)

The coronary arteries, which are responsible for supplying the heart with blood, are one of the main areas affected by the disease known as atherosclerosis. During physical exertion, when the heart requires more oxygen, the development of ischemia, or death to a tissue, may cause chest pain. This chest pain is called *angina pectoris*. This type of angina is classified as a vasospastic angina, often occurring when a patient is at rest. Its cause is due to vasospasms of the coronary arteries. The vasospasm decreases the blood flow, which may lead to myocardial ischemia.

Three major classifications of drugs are used in the treatment of angina. These include the nitrates and nitrites, beta-adrenergic blockers, and calcium antagonists.

Nitrates and Nitrites

Nitrates and nitrites are classified according to their administration during attacks of angina. They are used to relieve the intense pain, and their most common route of administration is sublingual, or under the tongue.

These drugs may also be administered prophylactically—that is, as a preventative measure in order to word off any future attacks of angina.

The five major nitrates and nitrites used in the treatment of angina pectoris include amyl nitrite, erythrityl tetranitrate, isosorbide dinitrate, nitroglycerin, and pentaerythritol tetranitrate. The most common adverse effect of these drugs is that they are related to the vasodilating action, and, consequently, may cause cutaneous flushing, dizziness, headache,

TABLE 12-4
Nitrites and Nitrates Used in Angina Pectoris

Drug Name	Dose	Onset	Duration
Amyl nitrite	0.3 ml inhalation	30–60 sec	10 min
Erythrityl tetranitrate	0–10 mg sublingual	5 min	3–4 hours
	10–25 mg P.O. QID	30 min	3–4 hours
Isosorbide dinitrate	5–10 mg sublingual	2–5 min	2–4 hours
	5–30 mg P.O. QID	30 min	2–4 hours
Nitroglycerin			
Nitrol	2% ointment	15 min	4–8 hours
Nitrostat	0.15–0.6 mg sublingual	1–3 min	10–45 min
Nitrong	2.6, 6.5, and 9.0 mg extend-release tablet	30 min	8–12 hours
Nitro-bid	2.5, 6.5, and 9.0 mg extend-release capsule	30–60 min	8–12 hours
Transderm-Nitro	2.5–15 mg/day transdermal patch	30–60 min	24 hours
Pentaerythritol tetranitrate	10–20 mg P.O. QID	30 min	3–4 hours

weakness, and fainting. Blood pressure usually decreases when these drugs are administered, and because of this they may cause a reflex tachycardia. Drugs classified in this category should never be used for patients who suffer from glaucoma, for vasodilation may increase intraoccular pressure in the eyes. (See Table 12–4.)

Beta Blockers

Beta blockers antagonize or reverse the effects of sympathetic activation caused by exercise and other physical or mental exertions. In the heart, sympathetic stimulation increases not only the heart rate but the force of myocardial contraction and oxygen consumption. Therefore, the

TABLE 12-5
Vasodilator Drugs Used in Congestive Heart Failure

Vasodilator	Main effect	Effect on heart
Captopril	Decreases formation of angiotensin and produces dilation of arteriolar and venous vessels	Increased cardiac output
Hydralazine	Dilates arteriolar more than venous vessels	Increased cardiac output
Nitroglycerin	Dilates venous more than arteriolar vessels	Decreased venous return and work of the heart
Prazosin	Dilates arteriolar and venous vessels	Increased cardiac output
Sodium nitroprusside	Dilates arteriolar and venous vessels	Increased cardiac output

therapeutic action of these drugs to treat angina lies in their ability to decrease the heart rate and the force of the contraction. These changes in turn decrease the cardiac work load and, therefore, oxygen consumption. The decreasing oxygen consumption often prevents the development of myocardial ischemia and pain.

Calcium Antagonists

Calcium antagonists interfere with the movement of calcium ions through the cell membranes. By doing so, they inhibit calcium influx and thereby decrease vascular tone, producing a vasodilating effect. The three calcium antagonists used in the treatment of angina are verapamil, diltiazem, and nifedipine. (See Table 12–5.)

UNDERSTANDING THE USE OF DIURETICS

The primary function of diuretics is to assist the kidneys in their maintenance of water, electrolytes, and acid-base balance by increasing the amount of urine being produced by the kidneys. In the cardiac patient it is extremely important that the balance among these three areas be maintained. Otherwise, cardiac output is diminished, and eventually the patient may go into congestive heart failure.

Many different types of diuretics are available for use in the treatment of cardiac disorders. They are, however, classified into four major categories according to their use and absorption in the body. These four categories are osmotic diuretics, thiazide diuretics, organic acid diuretics, and potassium-sparing diuretics.

Osmotic diuretics are compounds that can be filtered by the glomerulus of the kidney, but not reabsorbed by the renal tubules. The most commonly used of these include Diamox (trade name) and mannitol, with mannitol being the most frequently used by most cardiologists. Once inside the circulation, these drugs act osmotically, attracting fluid from edematous tissues, eventually causing diuresis. Mannitol is used primarily to stimulate the urine flow in the treatment of anuria, or lack of diuresis, and oliguria (acute renal failure). The major disadvantage of using osmotic diuretis is that, owing to their route of administration and low intensity of diuresis, there is a limit to their clinical use.

Thiazide diuretics have their therapeutic action on the renal tubules of the kidneys. These drugs are the most abundant in usage, and the most common include chlorothiazide (Diuril), chlorthalidone (Hygroton), and hydrochlorothiazide (HydroDIURIL). These drugs may be administered by mouth in order to produce a diuretic response. All of the drugs differ in their potency and duration of action; however, they all primarily produce diuresis by inhibiting the sodium transport in the distal portions of the nephrons located within the kidneys. (See Table 12–6.)

The third group of diuretics, referred to as *organic acid,* promote diuresis by inhibiting sodium and chloride transport in the loop of Henle, within the kidneys. The most commonly used drug in the treatment of cardiac patients is furosemide, or Lasix (trade name). Known as a "loop

TABLE 12–6
Recommended Doses of Thiazide and Thiazidelike Diuretics

Drug name (generic)	Duration of action (hr)	Adult oral dose (mg/day)
Thiazides		
Bendroflumethiazide	>18	5
Benzthiazide	12–18	50–200
Chlorothiazide	6–12	500–1,000
Cyclothiazide	18–24	1–2
Hydrochlorothiazide	6–12	50–100
Hydroflumethiazide	18–24	50–100
Methyclothiazide	>24	2.5–10
Polythiazide	24–48	1–4
Trichlormethiazide	24	1–4
Thiazidelike diuretics		
Chlorthalidone	24–72	50–100
Indapamide	up to 36	2.5–5
Metolazone	12–24	5–20
Quinethazone	18–24	50–100

diuretic," the drug causes an action that results in a tremendous loss of sodium, chloride, and water, eventually causing intense diuresis, usually accompanied by hypochloremic alkalosis.

The last group of diuretics used by many cardiac patients are termed (potassium-sparing). While their major disadvantage is the decrease of the electrolyte potassium—which if left untreated may throw the acid-base balance of all electrolytes of the body out of balance—they are also most useful, because of their oral route of administration. The most commonly used drugs in this group include amiloride hydrochloride (Moduretic), spironolactone (Aldactone), and triemterene (Dyrenium), with Aldactone being the most frequently used of the three. Following oral administration, these drugs produce diuresis by inhibiting potassium secretion in the distal convoluted tubules of the kidneys. All three drugs produce a mild diuresis without inducing electrolyte changes or imbalances in either the electrolytes or acid-base balance. (See Table 12–7.)

AGENTS/DIURETICS USED IN TREATING HYPERTENSION

Hypertension, a condition in which blood pressure in the arterial system is abnormally high, is one of the leading causes of cerebral strokes, heart attacks, and kidney disease. Approximately one-half of those who have hypertension are aware of their disease, but many of these people are not receiving proper treatment.

In the majority of hypertensive cases—about 90 percent—the cause of the disorder is not known. This type of hypertension is called *essential hypertension*. When the cause of the disorder is known, it is referred to as *secondary hypertension*. Since the basic cause of essential hypertension is unknown, the goal of drug therapy is aimed at lowering the blood pressure without causing excessive adverse effects on the patient.

TABLE 12-7
Organic-Acid and Potassium-Sparing Diuretics

Drug name	Use	Adult oral dose
Organic acids, Loop diuretics		
Ethacrynic acid	Edema associated with CHF, renal disease, and ascites (short-term)	50-100 mg/day
Furosemide	Edema associated with CHF, renal disease, and ascites (short-term)	20-80 mg/day
Potassium-sparing diuretics		
Amiloride and hydrochlorothiazide	Hypertension	1-2 tablets/day
Spironolactone	Hypertension	50-100 mg/day
	Edema	100-200 mg/day
	Hyperaldosteronism	100-400 mg/day
Spironolactone and hydrochlorothiazide	Hyperaldosteronism, Edema, hypertension	1-2 tablets/day
Triamterene	Edema	100-300 mg/day
Triamterene and hydrochlorothiazide	Edema, hypertension	1 or 2 capsules B.I.D.

The drugs used in the treatment of hypertension include diuretics, sympathetic or adrenergic blockers, vasodilators, and angiotension-converting enzymes. In advanced cases of hypertension, these drugs are used in combination with one another. It is important to note here that the pharmacological treatment of hypertension usually follows a certain sequence or steps, which are referred to as the "step-care" approach. In essence, what this means is that a drug listed in this classification is not given until another drug has already been tried and found not to be useful in the patient's treatment. Therefore, these "first" drugs are classified as "step 1" drugs.

Diuetics used in the treatment of hypertension include chlorothiazide, hydrochlorothiazide, methyclothiazide, and quinethazone. All act in such a way as to decrease the level of sodium being produced in the body by increasing the diuresis of urine production in the kidneys.

If the patient's blood pressure cannot be adequately controlled using step 1 drugs, he or she is ready to try medications classified as step 2 preparations. Known as *sympathetic blocking agents,* the most frequently used drugs in this category include reserpine, methyldopa, and prazosin. All of these are administered to the patient in order to decrease the overactive sympathetic nervous system and thereby interfere with the manufacture, storage, and release of norepinephrine. Less norepinephrine is available to produce vasoconstriction, and eventually, because of this, the blood pressure is reduced.

Step 3 drugs are introduced when the blood pressure has not been adequately controlled with the implementation of the drugs in steps 1 and 2. The step 3 medications include the vasodilators, with the most common ones being hydralazine and minoxidil. All of these drugs act directly on the smooth vascular muscle in order to cause relaxation. Vasodilation is then produced and the blood pressure is decreased.

If the blood pressure has not been adequately controlled with step-3 drugs, step 4 is introduced. This includes the use of the more potent sympathetic blockers, vasodilators or angiotension-converting enzyme inhibitors. Captopril, the only drug currently approved by the FDA for use as a step-4 antihypertensive agent, inhibits the enzymatic formation of angiotension in the blood.

UNDERSTANDING ANTICOAGULANTS AND COAGULANTS

When we discuss the drugs and medicinal preparations most frequently administered to patients suffering from disorders of the heart and cardiovascular system, it is important to address those medications that have a direct effect on the clotting mechanism taking place in the blood.

Clot formation is essential to human survival. Usually a blood clot acts as a seal that prevents any further loss of blood, oxygen, and nutrients from a wounded area. Anticoagulants are employed in the prevention of venous clotting in patients who have thromboembolic disorders, by interfering with the ability of the blood to form stable clots.

There are two classifications of anticoagulants most frequently used. These include the coumarinlike drugs and heparin. The coumarinlike anticoagulants prevent the synthesis of normal clotting factors. Anticoagulants, such as heparin, inhibit the function of the preformed clotting factors.

Heparin and the coumarinlike drugs are most commonly used in the prevention of venous thrombosis, especially pulmonary embolism. Therefore, these agents are normally used in the treatment of myocardial infarction, thrombophylebitis, and cerebral vascular accidents, or strokes.

Oral anticoagulants are usually considered the drugs of choice, for they are relatively inexpensive and can be taken quite easily by the patient. Heparin, on the other hand, is always the preferred drug when an anticoagulant must be given to a pregnant woman; this is because heparin does not cross the placenta and cannot affect the developing fetus. Also, because heparin cannot be given orally, and because it is destroyed by gastric acids, its administration parenterally—that is, by intravenous or subcutaneous injection—is almost always preferred because of its quick absorption into the blood.

The coumarin anticoagulants include dicumarol, phenprocoumon, and warfarin sodium. All of these are significantly different from heparin, and all can be administered orally. Of the three, warfarin sodium is usually considered the drug of choice.

Use of Vitamin K

There are times when an agent is required to decrease the incidence or severity of hemorrhage. In these cases, vitamin K and protamine sulfate, as specific antidotes for anticoagulant overdose, may be used as coagulants.

Another coagulant, called *aminocaproic acid,* can also be used as an inhibitor for the activation of fibrinolysin, in situations where fibrinosis (excessive fibrin in the blood) is present. Thrombin, which is obtained from cattle, is a direct activator of fibrin formation and will initiate clot formation when applied topically to actively oozing injuries. (See Table 12–8.)

TABLE 12–8
Commonly Used Anticoagulant Drugs

Drug name	Daily maintenance dose	Coagulation test employed
Dicumarol	25–200 mg p.O.	Prothrombin time
Diphenadione	3–5 mg P.O.	Prothrombin time
Heparin sodium	10,000–12,000 U every 12 hours S.C.	Whole-blood clotting time;
	5,000–10,000 U every 4–6 hours I.V.	Partial prothrombin time
Phenindione	50–150 mg P.O. BID	Prothrombin time
Phenprocoumon	0.75–6 mg P.O.	Prothrombin time
Warfarin sodium	2–10 mg P.O.	Prothrombin time

REVIEW QUESTIONS

Directions: For the questions below, give the answers you believe are most correct:

1. _____ _____ are primarily given to patients suffering from congestive heart failure.

2. The use of the drug _____ helps to increase the force of myocardial contraction during congestive heart failure.

3. _____ and _____ are two of the most widely used drugs for the treatment of congestive heart failure.

4. List at least three major adverse reactions caused by drugs given for the treatment of congestive heart failure:

   (a) _____

   (b) _____

   (c) _____

5. When are antiarrhythmic drugs administered?

6. Identify at least three Class I antiarrhythmic drugs:

   (a) _____

   (b) _____

   (c) _____

7. What is the name of the only Class II antiarrhythmic drug used as a beta blocker?

8. What is the name of the only Class III antiarrhythmic drug that may be used in the treatment of ventricular tachycardia?

9. Class IV antiarrhythmic drugs are also referred to as _____

   _____ _____ .

10. The administration of the Class IV antiarrhythmic drug _____

    _____ is most useful in the treatment of various types of AV nodal arrhythmias.

11. List the three major classifications of drugs used in the treatment of angina:

    (a) _____

    (b) _____

    (c) _____

12. What is the function of beta blockers?

13. What is the primary function of diuretics?

14. What are the four categories of diuretics?

    (a) _____

    (b) _____

    (c) _____

    (d) _____

15. Identify at least on diuretic used most often in the treatment of hypertension:

16. Administration of _____ and _____ has a direct effect on the clotting mechanism of the blood.

Cardiopulmonary Resuscitation

13

TERMINAL OBJECTIVE

To provide the student with an understanding of the principles and techniques involved in the performance of cardiopulmonary resuscitation.

COMPETENCY OBJECTIVES

Upon completion of this chapter, the student will be able to

1. Discuss the need for the EKG technician to learn and understand the principles and techniques involved in performing cardiopulmonary resuscitation (CPR).
2. Explain the purpose of an EMS system.
3. Discuss and demonstrate how to perform rescue breathing on an adult victim.
4. Discuss and demonstrate how to care for both a conscious and an unconscious adult victim who has an obstructed airway.
5. Discuss and demonstrate how to perform one-rescuer CPR on an adult victim.
6. Discuss how to deal with respiratory emergencies in infants and children.
7. Explain how to check the consciousness of an infant or child suspected of respiratory arrest.
8. Discuss and demonstrate how to care for an infant or child who has an obstructed airway.
9. Discuss and demonstrate how to perform CPR on an infant or child.

GUIDELINES

As a member of the cardiology team, the EKG technician may be called upon at any given time to administer the techniques involved in cardio-pulmonary resuscitation, or CPR*. Therefore, it is extremely important that you understand the principles and skills involved in performing CPR, including those techniques associated with rescue breathing, dealing with an obstructed airway, and performing these techniques on adults, children, and infants.

In June 1986 the *Journal of the American Medical Association* published new guidelines for teaching cardiopulmonary resuscitation. Prior to this, members of the American Red Cross, American Heart Association, and the Lung and Blood Institute met to sponsor a conference in which 300 medical practitioners and emergency care providers developed these standards. Their primary goal was to simplify and standardize CPR instruction for the general public.

While information being provided at this time is considered to be up-to-date and standardized, the EKG technician should also understand that new principles and techniques for providing emergency cardiopulmonary resuscitation to the victim is continuously being revised and altered so as to ensure that the optimal techniques in life-saving skills are being practiced throughout the world.

EMERGENCY MEDICAL SERVICES (EMS) SYSTEM

An emergency medical services, or EMS, system is a communitywide, coordinated means of responding to an accident or sudden illness. It is a method in which we bring all members of society into a system of caring for the life-threatened victim.

An EMS system is composed of three parts: entry into the system, rescue and transportation, and hospital emergency facilities.

*Author's disclaimer: It is important for the reader to understand that the information presented in this chapter deals with certain techniques and methods that may be utilized during the course of saving a victim's life, as in the case of a cardiac arrest. Both the American Red Cross and the American Heart Association continually work together in revising and redefining new methods of ensuring that victims receive the best and most crucial first aid available during the first few moments in which cardiopulmonary resuscitation (CPR) may be initiated. Therefore, it is also important to note that, while the material presented in this chapter meets the most up-to-date guidelines recommended by both the American Red Cross and the American Heart Association for performing cardiopulmonary resuscitation and rescue-breathing, the author suggests that the reader contact his or her local Red Cross or American Heart office to obtain any additional information regarding changes in CPR methodology.

Entry Into the System

Two kinds of action are needed to enter a victim into the EMS system. The first is through bystanders providing immediate emergency care. This greatly increases the survival chances of a victim of an accident or sudden illness. As many people as possible should be trained in first aid and CPR.

The second action occurs at the same time, or as soon as possible, in which another bystander "activates the EMS system." This includes phoning 911 or dialing the operator or the local EMS number.

Whenever someone calls for emergency help, that person should remember to provide the person taking the call with the following information:

1. WHERE the emergency situation is.
2. PHONE NUMBER you are calling from.
3. WHAT HAPPENED? Heart attack? Auto accident? Etc.
4. HOW MANY people need help?
5. YOU HANG UP LAST! Let the person you called hang up first.

Rescue and Transportation

Upon receiving the emergency call, a trained professional may be sent to the scene in order to provide more definitive care. These individuals bring with them knowledge, expertise, and the necessary tools to rescue, stabilize, and transport the victim.

Hospital Emergency Facilities

At the hospital, further stabilizing care is provided and medical procedures begun by physicians, nurses, and technicians. However, all of the sophisticated equipment and specialized training available at an emergency facility will be of little value if immediate care has not been given at the scene and the EMS system not activated.

RESCUE BREATHING: ADULT VICTIM

During a respiratory emergency, all breathing either ceases or is so reduced that the victim is not able to take in enough oxygen to support life. Causes of respiratory failure include heart attack, stroke, drowning, airway obstruction by a foreign object, the tongue, or food; circulatory collapse caused by shock or hemorrhaging; overdose of drugs or other toxins; electrocution, toxic gases, suffocation, and external strangulation, as in hanging.

Rescue breathing allows for the flow of air in and out of the lungs of a person whose breathing has either stopped or has become inadequate. During the rescue breathing process, it is the rescuer who forces air from his or her lungs into the victim's lungs.

Air that is inhaled contains approximately 21 percent oxygen, and air that is exhaled contains about 16 percent oxygen. In air that you exhale, enough oxygen remains to support life. As long as the other life-supporting functions are still working, rescue breathing will keep the victim alive.

Assessing the Victim

Assessing the victim involves three phases, or what is most commonly referred to as "checking the A, B, Cs."

A stands for airway. If the victim is unresponsive, call for help, then tilt the victim's head in order to open the airway.

B stands for breathing. Check to see if the victim is breathing. If breathing has stopped, give the victim two breaths.

C stands for circulation. This means you must check the victim's pulse. If no pulse, start chest compressions. Also activate the EMS system.

Checking for Consciousness

If someone suddenly collapses you will need to find out right away if he or she is conscious. This is accomplished through "tapping" the victim's shoulder firmly or shaking the victim gently and shouting, "Are you OK?" A victim who is conscious will respond and will not have stopped breathing. Make sure you look for other problems and keep checking for consciousness. Never shake the person vigorously if there is any possibility of a neck or back injury.

If the victim does not respond, you must shout "Help!" in order to get the attention of others who may be able to assist you.

Positioning the Victim

If the victim is unconscious you will need to check for breathing and, depending upon the person's condition, you may have to give rescue breathing, correct a blocked airway, or administer CPR. The victim must be lying on his or her back in order to initiate CPR, and rescue breathing is facilitated if the victim is also lying on his or her back.

If the victim is lying face down, or in some other awkward position, you must consider injuries you might cause or make worse by moving the victim.

If you are sure that the victim collapsed without injuries, you will need to position the person on his or her back immediately. If you are caring for a victim of a violent accident, however, it is better to check for breathing before moving the victim at all. In most cases, you will have to rely on your best judgment.

If you find you have to move the victim, your goal should be to roll the person as one unit, all at once, without twisting any body parts. You may do this by first straightening the victim's arms and legs so that they won't get in the way. Then roll the victim toward you, onto his or her back, and support the head and neck with one hand, pulling with the other just under the victim's arm. Remember to keep the body from twisting.

Always check the breathing of an unconscious person right away. Remember, you have only a few minutes to save the life of someone whose breathing has stopped, and every moment you wait makes recovery less likely. Permanent brain damage may occur very quickly, sometimes in less time than 4 minutes.

The Airway Step

The first steps involved in caring for an unconscious person entail determining unresponsiveness, calling for help, then opening the victim's airway by tilting back the victim's head. You must remember to tilt the person's head way back, until the chin points straight up. By doing so, the head moves the lower jaw forward, and because the tongue is attached to the lower jaw, tilting in this manner opens the airway. If tilting is not performed, the tongue may block the airway.

Head-Tilt With Chin Lift

Place one hand on the victim's forehead and apply firm, backward pressure with the palm of the hand. This is considered the major force in tilting the head. To help move the tongue away from the back of the throat, place the fingertips of your other hand under the bony part of the jaw near the chin. Then support and lift the lower jaw with your fingertips, making sure you avoid closing the victim's mouth. The victim's chin should point straight up.

There are five important points to remember when performing the head-tilt chin lift. They are:

1. Apply the major force with your hand on the victim's forehead;
2. place your fingertips under the bony part of the victim's jaw near the chin;
3. support and lift the victim's jaw with your fingertips, but make sure you avoid closing the victim's mouth;
4. never push on the soft tissues of the throat as this may block the victim's airway;
5. if necessary, pull the victim's lower lip down slightly with your thumb in order to keep the victim's mouth open.

The Breathing Step

As you begin to tilt the victim's head and lift the chin, you should put your ear down near the mouth of the victim and examine the victim's chest. Look, listen, and feel for breathing for approximately 3 to 5 seconds. If the person is breathing, you will see the chest rise and fall, hear air at the mouth and nose, and feel air on your cheek. If the person is not breathing, you must immediately give two full slow breaths to the victim.

When performing the breathing step, you must remember to always keep the victim's head tilted. Pinch the victim's nose so air will not come out when you blow into the victim's mouth. Take a deep breath and open your mouth wide. Cover the victim's mouth with your own, making sure you provide a good seal. Give two full slow breaths, taking about 1 to $1\frac{1}{2}$ seconds for each breath. Remove your mouth from the victim's mouth between breaths long enough to allow the lungs to deflate. (See Figure 13–1.)

The Circulation Step

After you have given the victim two full slow breaths, check the victim's pulse. This is accomplished by checking the pulse on the side of the neck near you, or what we refer to as "over the carotid artery." Keep the victim's head tilted with your hand on the victim's forehead. Place the fingertips of your other hand on the victim's Adam's apple, then slide your fingers into the groove at the side of the neck. Make sure you check the pulse for at least 5 seconds, but never more than 10 seconds.

If the victim is not breathing, but does have a pulse, give rescue breathing. If there is no breathing and no pulse, CPR will need to be started immediately. In either case, the EMs system should be activated. The victim's heart may be beating even though you did not find a pulse, so rescue breathing may keep the person alive. (See Figure 13–2.)

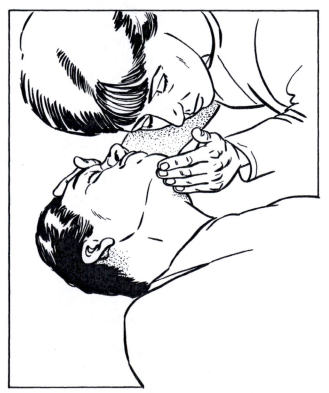

Figure 13–1   The breathing step.

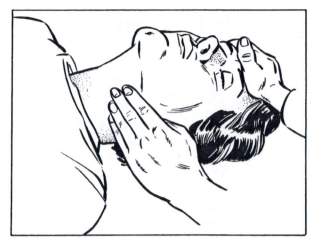

Figure 13–2   The circulation step.

Mouth-to-Nose Breathing

There may be times when it is impossible for you to make a good seal over the victim's mouth in order to perform rescue breathing. If this is indeed the case, you will need to initiate mouth-to-nose breathing. To do this, you should

1. tilt the head, using the chin-lift;
2. close the victim's mouth and push on the chin, not the throat, so that you do not shut the victim's airway;
3. blow into the victim's nose;
4. open the victim's mouth and listen for air; watch the chest fall. (See Figure 13–3.)

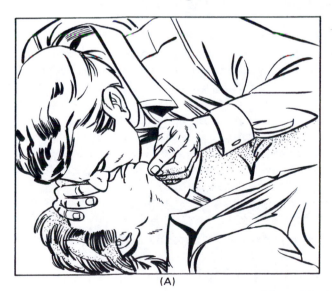

(A)

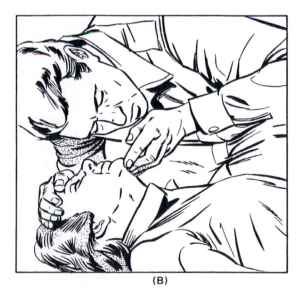

(B)

Figure 13–3   Mouth-to-nose breathing.

Air in the Stomach

When administering rescue breathing, the victim's stomach may fill up with air. If this occurs, the air can push against the lungs, making it difficult or almost impossible to give full breaths. The air can be expelled by pushing on the victim's stomach; however, this is considered dangerous, for the victim may vomit or inhale the vomit into the lungs. When you give the breaths, try to blow just hard enough to make the chest rise; this way you will be less likely to force air into the victim's stomach.

If the victim's stomach appears to be distended or bulging with air and you are unable to inflate the victim's lungs, you should follow the steps below:

1. Turn the victim onto one side.
2. Push on the victim's stomach with your hand between the rib cage and the waist.
3. Clean out the mouth if the victim vomits.
4. Roll the victim onto his or her back and continue rescue breathing.

Remember, these steps should only be taken if air in the stomach prevents you from giving breaths.

Mouth-to-Stoma Breathing

There are approximately 25,000 people in the United States who have had all or part of their larynx, or voice box, removed by surgery. These people breathe through an opening in the front of the neck, called a *stoma*. If breathing has ceased on a victim who has a stoma, you will be required to perform mouth-to-stoma breathing.

A person with a stoma may have a passage from the lungs to the mouth and nose, so you may need to block the mouth and nose when you blow into the stoma. If the lungs do not inflate when administering air into the stoma, block the victim's mouth and nose with your hand.

If a person is wearing a breathing tube in the stoma and the tube becomes clogged, it is safe to remove it with the fingers in order to open the airway. If this is the case, remember to send the tube with the victim to the hospital, or allow the victim to clean and replace the tube. You should never try to replace the tube.

To administer mouth-to-stoma breathing, do the following:

1. Do not tilt the victim's head. Instead, keep the head and neck straight.
2. Check breathing with your ear near the stoma.
3. Give breaths with your mouth sealed over the stoma.
4. Block the victim's mouth and nose if air escapes from them when you blow into the stoma. (See Figure 13–4.)

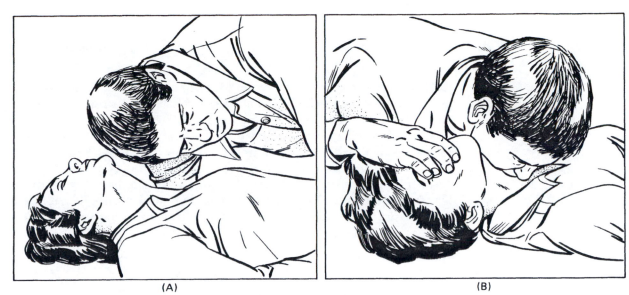

| (A) | (B) |

Figure 13-4 Mouth-to-stoma breathing.

Airway Obstruction

Two types of airway obstructions can inhibit the victim from receiving air. The first, called an *anatomic obstruction,* is caused by the tongue dropping back and blocking the throat, or by tissues in the throat swelling and interfering with breathing. Narrowing of the airway may be caused by disease, burns, or injury.

In an anatomical obstruction, tilting the victim's head will generally open the airway. If you cannot inflate the victim's lungs when you try to give breaths, retilt the victim's head and try again. You may not have tilted the head far enough the first time.

The second type of airway obstruction, called a *mechanical obstruction,* is a blockage of the airway that is caused by an object or by fluids such as mucous, blood, saliva, or vomit collecting in the back of the throat. Food is the most common mechanical obstruction in adults.

Choking on food may be caused in a number of ways, such as in the consumption of too much alcohol, which tends to cause a deadened sensation in the mouth. False teeth may also reduce normal sensations in the mouth, as can large bites of poorly chewed food. Surprisingly, large pieces of unchewed food are found blocking the throats of people who have choked to death.

The tongue and fluids such as blood or vomit are more likely to block the airway of an unconscious person who is lying flat on the back. Most people who need rescue breathing do not have a foreign object blocking the airway. Remember, if you cannot get air to go into the lungs, retilt the victim's head and try again to give the breaths. If that still does not work, it is most likely that an object may be blocking the person's airway.

Jutting the Jaw

If a person was in an accident and there is reason to suspect that he or she may have a broken neck or back, or that the bones in the face may be broken, you should never tilt the victim's head. Instead, you may be able to give breaths after pushing forward the victim's jaw—that is, jutting or thrusting the jaw without tilting the victim's head. To accomplish this, place your fingers on the corners of the person's jaw and push the jaw forward. Keep the jaw forward as you give the breaths, letting your cheek puff out to block the victim's nose when you blow. (See Figure 13–5.)

If the victim's head, face, neck, or back has been injured and you are unable to inflate the person's lungs with the head straight and the jaw forward, it may be necessary to tilt the victim's head as a last resort. To do this, tilt it only slightly, just enough to allow you to inflate the injured person's lungs.

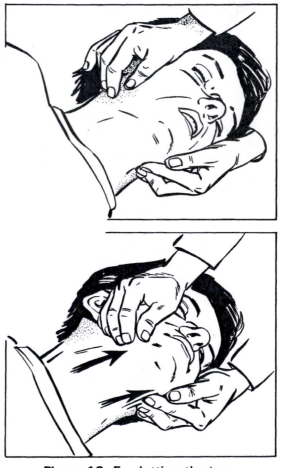

Figure 13–5   Jutting the jaw.

ONE-RESCUER CPR: ADULT VICTIM

The heart and the lungs work together. Air that is inhaled into the lungs provides oxygen to the blood. The heart circulates the blood, carrying oxygen to the brain and to the rest of the body. If a person stops breathing, the heart may keep beating for a short time. If this is the case, rescue breathing should be initiated immediately. However, if a heart attack, illness, or injury, causes the heart to stop beating, or what we refer to as *cardiac arrest,* breathing will not continue. In this case, cardio-pulmonary resuscitation, or CPR, must be started.

In cardiopulmonary resuscitation, *cardio* refers to the heart and *pulmonary* refers to the lungs. CPR is the combination of rescue breathing, which supplies the oxygen to the lungs, and chest compressions, which circulate the blood. By administering CPR, you in fact are breathing and circulating blood for another person whose heart and lungs have stopped working.

SIGNALS OF A HEART ATTACK

In Chapter 9 we discussed myocardial infarctions, or what we commonly refer to as a heart attack, in great depth. You should note, however, that the most typical signals indicating that someone is having a heart attack include feelings of uncomfortable pressure, squeezing, fullness, or pain in the center of the chest. Sometimes the pain is in the upper abdomen, causing the victim to feel like he or she is experiencing indigestion. Pain may also travel out from the center of the chest, to the shoulders, arms, neck, and jaw. Other signals may include diaphoreis, or profuse sweating, nausea, shortness of breath, and a general feeling of weakness.

Anyone who is experiencing persistent signals of an impending heart attack should get medical care at once. This may mean calling the paramedics or rescue squad or taking the person to a hospital right away.

Factors Influencing a Heart Attack

A number of factors are either known to increase the risk of a heart attack or are strongly suspected of contributing to the risk of one. These include hypertension, obesity, smoking, vigorous exercise not normally undertaken, and increased intake of saturated fats and cholesterol in the diet. Many of these factors work together, such as obesity, hypertension, and poor nutritional habits. Having regular checkups to identify possible risk factors, such as high blood pressure and obesity, will decrease a person's risk of an impending heart attack.

PERFORMING CPR

Chest Compressions

As we have already noted, CPR is the combination of rescue breathing and chest compressions. Chest compressions are responsible for circulating the blood by pressing the heart between the sternum, or breastbone, and the backbone. The sternum runs down the front of the chest, and the ribs join it in the front at a structure known as the *xiphoid process.*

When you administer chest compressions, you push on the lower half of the sternum, just above the xiphoid process. Never push directly

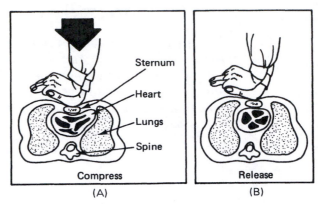

Figure 13-6   Chest compressions.

on this structure; doing so may cause injury to the victim. (See Figure 13-6.)

Deciding Where to Give Chest Compressions

To decide where to give chest compressions you must first find the lower edge of the victim's rib cage on the side nearest you. Use your hand that is nearer the victim's feet. With your middle and index fingers, trace the edge of the ribs up to the notch where the ribs meet the sternum. This is the center of the lower chest.

Keep your middle finger on the notch and place your index finger next to it on the lower end of the sternum. Put the heel of your other hand on the sternum, next to your fingers. If you by accident push on the xiphoid process it may bend in and injure the liver. It is better to be too high on the sternum rather than to be too low.

Next put your other hand on top of the hand on the sternum, making sure to keep your fingers off the victim's chest. You are more likely to break a rib if you push with your fingers, so you may either lace your fingers, holding them up, or grasp them with the wrist of your other hand. You are now ready to begin chest compressions. (See Figure 13-7.)

Administering Chest Compressions

"Stand" on your knees, and do not sit on your heels. Place your knees about a shoulder-width apart. With your shoulders directly over the victim's sternum, and your hands along the middle line of your body, push straight down. Use your body weight, and make sure to keep your elbows straight.

When you push, bend from your hips, not your knees. This makes it easier to push straight down. If you start to rock back and forth on your knees, you will not be pushing correctly.

With your fingers pointing across the victim's chest away from you, push straight down. Compress the chest of an adult $1\frac{1}{2}$ to 2 inches. Push very smoothly, and do not jerk. Keep your hands resting lightly on the victim's chest between compressions.

Compress the chest at a rate of 80 to 100 compressions per minute when giving one-rescuer CPR to an adult. As you give the compressions,

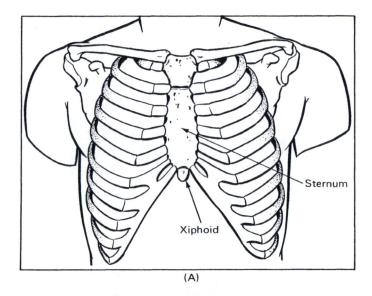

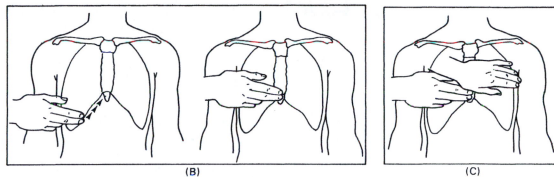

Figure 13-7 Deciding where to give chest compressions.

count aloud, "One-and, two-and, three-and," and so forth, while you are learning and practicing. (See Figure 13-8.)

When you administer CPR, the victim's head should be at the level of the heart or slightly lower than the heart. If the victim's head is higher, blood will not flow to the brain.

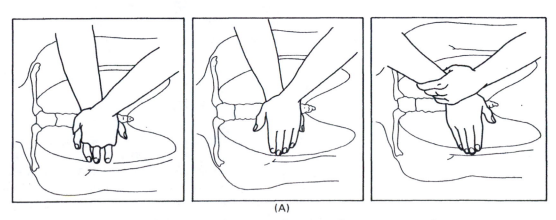

Figure 13-8 Administering chest compressions.

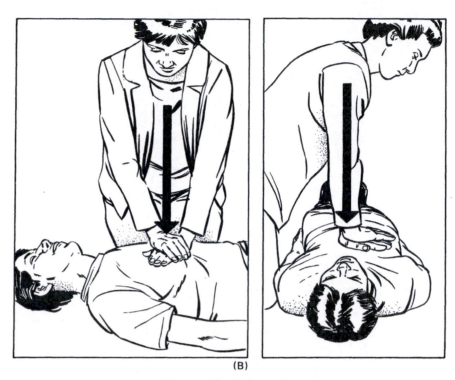

(B)

Figure 13-8 (cont.)

Remember to make sure that the victim is lying on a firm surface. If he or she is lying on a soft bed or in the water, chest compressions will not press the heart between the backbone and the sternum.

As soon as possible, elevate the feet and legs of the victim. This helps the blood return to the heart. Remember, do not stop giving CPR to elevate the legs; have another person do it.

Combining Chest Compressions and Rescue Breathing

In one-rescuer CPR, you must give 15 compressions at the rate of 80 to 100 per minute. This is followed by 2 full breaths, 1 to $1\frac{1}{2}$ seconds each. Keep repeating 15 compressions, 2 breaths; 15 compressions, 2 breaths. . . . And each time you begin the 15 compressions, remember to measure up quickly from the notch where the ribs meet the sternum. (See Figure 13-9.)

OBSTRUCTED AIRWAY: CONSCIOUS ADULT VICTIM

If you see someone choking on food or suspect that a person is choking if he or she collapses while eating, there is a very good possibility that person is suffering from an obstructed airway. Conscious victims may show signs of an obstructed airway through difficult breathing. Signs of difficulty include wheezing, gasping, choking, coughing, and grasping the throat.

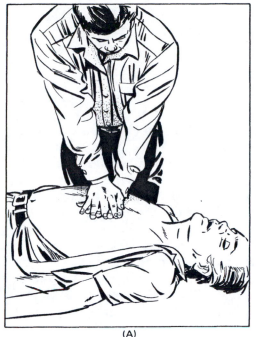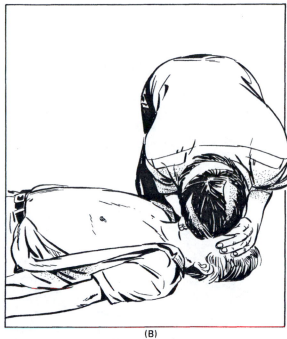

(A)   (B)

Figure 13–9   Administering one-rescuer CPR to an adult.

If the person is not coughing, ask, "Are you choking?" A person who has a completely blocked airway cannot breathe, cough, or speak.

If the airway is almost completely blocked, there may be high-pitched noises when inhaling, great difficulty breathing, and very weak or no coughing. First aid is the same for a completely blocked airway as it is for one that is almost completely blocked.

Someone who is coughing forcefully should be left entirely alone. Watch closely and encourage the person to cough. Normal coughing is more effective than any mechanical method taught for opening an obstructed airway.

If the person can speak, do not try to remove an object from the airway.

Conscious Choking Victim

If the victim is unable to speak, cough, or breathe, you should call for help and then give abdominal thrusts. Abdominal thrusts, or what we refer to as the *Heimlich maneuver*, is administered in the midline of the abdomen, slightly above the navel, and well below the tip of the xiphoid process. Never push on the edge of the rib cage or on the xiphoid process; this may injure the victim.

To administer abdominal thrusts, make a fist and put the thumb side against the victim's navel. Grasp your fist with your other hand and press it into the victim's abdomen with a quick inward and upward thrust. Do not exert pressure against the victim's rib cage. Each thrust should be distinct and delivered with the intent of relieving the airway obstruction. Repeat the thrusts until the object is expelled or the victim becomes unconscious. (See Figure 13-10.)

Unconscious Choking Victim

Should the victim lose consciousness, you must attempt to assist the person to the floor without injuring yourself or the victim. Position the victim on the back, face up. Call for help again, or if others respond, direct them to activate the EMS system.

Immediately perform a *finger sweep*. This is accomplished by grasping the victim's tongue and lower jaw between your thumb and fingers, and pulling up. With the index finger of your other hand, follow down along the inside of one cheek, deep into the throat to the base of the tongue. Sweep in from the side, and do not poke straight in, since that may push the object down. Use a hooking action, across toward the other cheek, to loosen and remove the object. (See Figure 13-11.)

Once you have completed the finger sweep, you must then attempt to ventilate the victim. If the airway remains blocked after you have retilted the head, perform abdominal thrusts. Straddle the victim's thighs, then put the heel of one hand on the victim's abdomen, in the midline slightly above the navel and well below the xiphoid process. Then put the other hand on top of the first hand. Point the fingers of the bottom hand toward the victim's head. With your shoulders directly over the

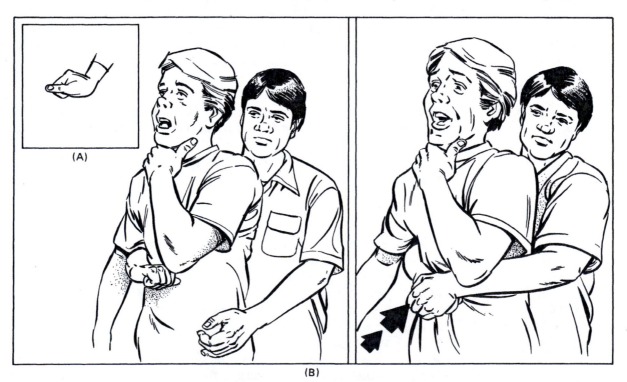

(A)

(B)

Figure 13-10 (A) Hand position for application of abdominal thrust for conscious choking victim; (B) application of Heimlich maneuver.

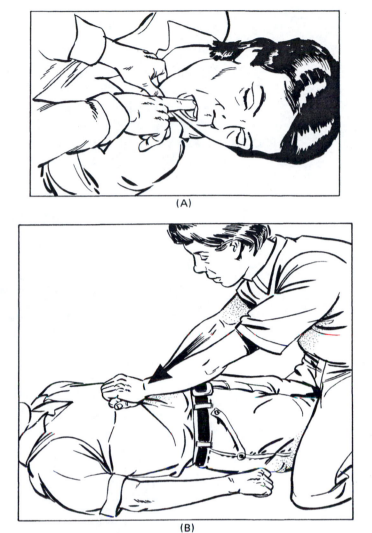

(A)

(B)

Figure 13-11 (A) Finger sweep for unconscious choking victim; (B) application of abdominal thrusts for unconscious choking victim.

victim's abdomen, press inward and upward with 6 to 10 abdominal thrusts. Do not press to either side; this may injure the victim.

Once you have completed the 6 to 10 abdominal thrusts, move back to the victim's head and perform a finger sweep, attempt to ventilate, and, if air still does not go in, perform another series of 6 to 10 abdominal thrusts. You should repeat this sequence until successful.

Chest Thrusts: Conscious Choking Victim

If the victim is in advanced pregnancy or so obese that you cannot reach around the waist, you should administer chest thrusts, not abdominal thrusts.

To perform chest thrusts on a conscious choking victim, you should do the following:

1. Reach around the chest from behind, with your arms directly under the victim's axilla (armpits).
2. Place the thumb side of your fist on the middle of the sternum at about the level of the axilla.
3. Grasp your fist with your other hand, and pull straight back with quick thrusts. (See Figure 13–12.)

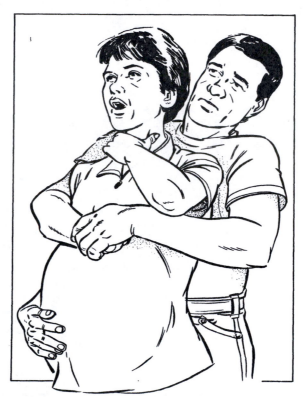

Figure 13–12   Application of chest thrusts for conscious choking victim.

RESPIRATORY EMERGENCIES: INFANTS AND CHILDREN

The most frequent accidental cause of respiratory emergencies in infants (children under the age of one) is choking, in which the airway becomes blocked by food or a foreign object. The disorder known as Sudden Infant Death Syndrome (SIDS), in which the infant stops breathing and its heart stops beating for some unknown reason, is also responsible for many of the respiratory emergencies encountered in infants.

Rescue breathing, CPR, and first aid for an obstructed airway are similar for both adults and children; however, some adaptations are required for the smaller sizes and faster breathing and heartbeats of youngsters. In defining methods used on young people, we will term anyone under one year of age an "infant" or "baby," and anyone between the ages of one and eight will be referred to as a "child." Methods for adults should be used on those children eight years of age and older. Remember, in an emergency your best bet is to use your own best judgment and never try to be exact about determining the victim's age, since a slight difference will not be critical.

Assessment

To remember the first steps for assessment of an infant or child victim, just as with an adult, we check the A, B, Cs. *A* pertains to airway. If unresponsive, call for help, then tilt the victim's head to open the airway. *B* is for breathing. If breathing is not noted, give two breaths. *C* is for circulation. Check the victim's pulse, activate the EMS system, and, if no pulse, begin chest compressions.

Checking Consciousness

You should check the consciousness of an infant or child in the same manner you did for an adult: Tap or gently shake a baby or child or shout, "Are you OK?"

Open the Airway

Put a hand on the victim's forehead and use the chin-lift to tilt the youngster's head back gently, but not as far as with an adult.

The Breathing Step

Look, listen, and feel for breathing for 3 to 5 seconds by putting your ear down close to the mouth and looking at the victim's chest. If there is no breathing, keep the victim's head tilted, open your mouth wide, and put it over the mouth and nose of the infant or child. If the child is too large for you to make a good seal over the mouth and nose, pinch the nose and make a seal over the mouth, as you would for an adult.

Give the youngster two slow, gentle breaths, at a rate of 1 to $1\frac{1}{2}$ seconds each. A gentle breath is defined as enough air to make the chest rise; allow for chest deflation after each ventilation.

The Circulation Step

After the breathing step, do the circulation step. Check the pulse of the child with your fingertips on the inside of the upper arm. This is accomplished by placing the tips of two fingers halfway between the elbow and the shoulder and placing your thumb on the opposite side of the arm and squeezing gently. Check the pulse of a child at the neck, just as you did for the adult, for at least 5 seconds, but no more than 10 seconds. (See Figure 13–13.)

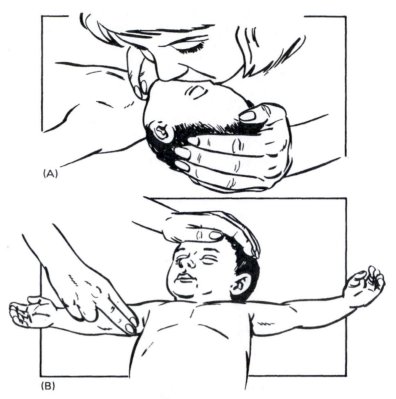

Figure 13-13 (A) Opening the infant's airway: the breathing step; (B) the circulation step.

If the infant is not breathing but does have a pulse, give mouth-to-mouth and nose breathing. Administer one slow gentle breath every 3 seconds, faster than for an adult. You can count, "One, one-thousand, two, one-thousand, b-r-e-a-t-h-e."

For a child, you will administer a breath every 4 seconds—that is, slower than for an infant but faster than for an adult. When you open the airway, the victim may struggle to breathe, or breathe weakly. If the victim does not seem to be getting enough oxygen, give breaths. Time your breaths with the victim's efforts to breathe. One sign of insufficient oxygen is blue lips.

If the victim is not breathing and does not have a pulse, CPR must be started immediately. Begin by initiating the EMS system. When you begin to give breaths, and the victim's stomach appears to be filling up with air—which occurs more frequently in infants and children than with adults—it may be a sign that you are blowing too hard or you may be dealing with a partially blocked airway. If this seems to be the case, check that the victim's head is tilted and that you are not blowing too hard. If air in the victim's stomach prevents you from giving breaths, take the following steps:

1. Turn the victim on one side.
2. Push on the victim's stomach with your hand between the rib cage and the waist.

3. Clean out the mouth if the victim vomits.

4. Roll the victim onto the back and continue rescue breathing.

Infant/Child Airway Obstruction

Like adults, infants and children may suffer from one of two types of airway obstructions. In the first type, the *anatomical* obstruction, the tongue can block the airway of an infant or small child just as it can block an adult's airway. If air will not go into the lungs, retilt the victim's head and try again. You can block a baby's airway by tilting the head too far, so tilt the head only a moderate amount.

In the second type of airway obstruction, called *mechanical*, you will be unable to inflate the victim's lungs until such time as you retilt the head and allow the airway to become unblocked by an object.

Removing a Foreign Object: Infant Victim

The basic steps for removing an object from the airway of an infant are different from those for an adult or child. If the infant is conscious, back blows and chest thrusts should be used. If the infant is unconscious, breaths, back blows, chest thrusts, and mouth sweep should be used if the object is visible.

Back Blows

To administer back blows to an infant, place the baby face down, straddling your arm, with the youngster's head lower than the chest. Support the head with your hand around the jaw and under the chest. Rest your arm on your thigh and apply the back blows rapidly between the shoulder blades with the heel of your hand. (See Figure 13–14.)

Turning the Infant Over

Place your free hand on the infant's back and sandwich the victim between your hands and arms. One hand supports the chest, neck, and jaw, and the other hand supports the back, neck, and head. Holding the baby between your hands and arms, turn it face up. Rest your arm on your thigh so that the infant's head is lower than the chest.

Chest Thrusts: Infant Victim

Push on the chest four times with two to three fingertips in the midsternal region, one finger-width below an imaginary line between the nipples. Your hand should come in from the side so that your fingertips run up and down the sternum, not across it.

If the infant is unconscious, think, "Breaths, blows, thrusts, look in the mouth." If you see an object, sweep the mouth.

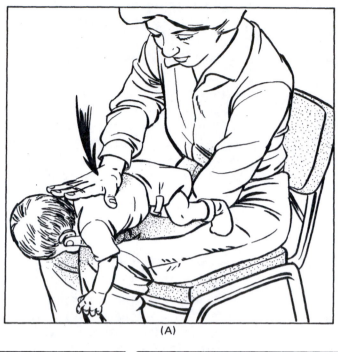

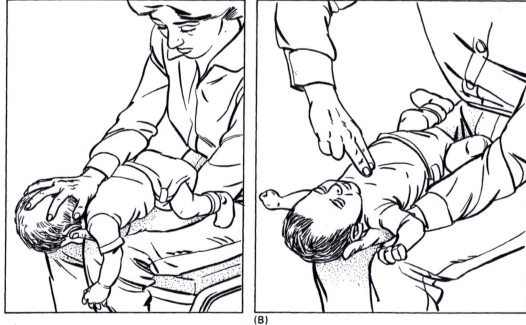

Figure 13–14 (A) Application of back blows on infant victim; (B) turning the infant over.

Finger Sweep

To perform a finger sweep, place your thumb in the mouth on the tongue and place your fingers around the chin. Lift the jaw and look in the mouth. If you see an object, remove it with a finger. Do not poke straight in;

rather, sweep in from the side. Because an infant or child has a small mouth, it is easy to push an object farther down by sweeping. Do not sweep unless you see the object.

Give Breaths

Whether or not you see an object and remove it, continue with the sequence, starting with "tilt the head and lift the chin." If the victim begins to breathe when you tilt the head to give breaths, stop giving first aid for choking, but keep watching to be sure the victim keeps on breathing. If the victim is not breathing when you tilt the head to do the airway step, try to give breaths. If you can inflate the lungs, give 2 slow, gentle breaths, and do the circulation step. If the heart is beating, keep giving rescue breathing. If the heart is not beating, CPR must be started. If the air will not go into the lungs, repeat 4 back blows, 4 thrusts, and a finger sweep if you can see an object. Then try again to give the breaths. Remember—keep trying!

Removing a Foreign Object: Child Victim

To remove a foreign body obstruction from a child, follow the same steps as for an adult victim, with one exception: Be sure you can see the object before doing a finger sweep.

If the child victim is conscious, administer abdominal thrusts (Heimlich maneuver), and if the child becomes unconscious, administer breaths, thrusts, and sweep the mouth, but only if you can see an object.

CPR FOR INFANTS AND CHILDREN

Chest Compressions: Infant Victim

Perform compressions on the infant one finger-width below the imaginary nipple line. To do this, place your index finger between the infant's nipples, your middle and ring fingers beside the index finger, and compress with the right and middle fingers. Never push on the lower end of the sternum (xiphoid process) as it can bend in and damage the liver.

To administer chest compressions do the following:

1. Compress a baby's chest $\frac{1}{2}$ inch to 1 inch.
2. Push smoothly and gently at least 100 times per minute. This is approximately twice a second.
3. Be sure that the victim's head is at the same level as the heart or slightly lower than the heart. If the victim's head is higher than the heart, chest compressions will not pump enough blood up to the brain.
4. Support the infant's back with one hand if tilting the head raises the back or if the infant is not on a firm surface. This will also help

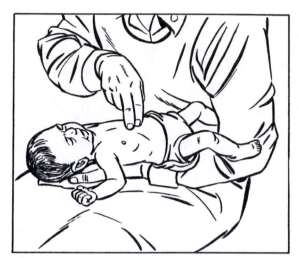

Figure 13-15 Application of chest compressions on infant victim.

keep the head tilted, ready for you to give a breath. (See Figure 13-15.)

Chest Compressions: Child Victim

Compress a child's chest with the heel of one hand. The proper hand position is located in a similar place to that used on an adult. Trace the edge of the ribs up to the notch where the ribs meet the sternum. This is considered the center of the lower chest.

Keep one finger on the notch and place another finger near it to measure one finger-width up from the notch, on the lower end of the sternum. Put the heel of one hand on the sternum at this location. (See Figure 13-16.)

Compress at a rate of 80 to 100 times per minute. Compress the chest a little more than you would a baby's chest, approximately 1 to

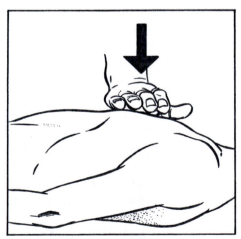

Figure 13-16 Application of chest compressions on child victim.

$1\frac{1}{2}$ inches. To help you time the rate of 80 to 100 compressions per minute, say, "One-and, two-and, three-and," and so forth.

Combining Chest Compressions and Breaths

The ratio of compressions to breaths is the same for both infants and children, namely five to one (5:1).

Give one breath after every fifth compression, pausing $1\frac{1}{2}$ seconds for ventilation. (See Table 13–1.)

If you are giving CPR, after every fifth compression open the airway and give one slow, gentle breath. Supporting an infant's back with one hand will help keep the head tilted, ready for the breath. Keep your face very close to the infant's face; this helps make it easier to give a breath quickly.

TABLE 13–1
CPR at a Glance

	Compression and Ventilation Reference Guide			
	Ventilation rate (one every)	*Compression-ventilation ratio*	*Compression rate (per minute)*	*Compression depth (inches)*
ADULT	5 seconds	15:2	80–100	$1\frac{1}{2}$–2
CHILD	4 seconds	5:1	80–100	1–$1\frac{1}{2}$
INFANT	3 seconds	5:1	at least 100	$\frac{1}{2}$–1

REVIEW QUESTIONS

Directions: For the questions below, give the answers you believe are most correct:

1. What are the three parts of the airway step?

    (a) _____

    (b) _____

    (c) _____

2. How do you check to see if a victim is breathing?

3. How long do you check for breathing?

4. On an adult, when checking for circulation, where do you find the pulse?

5. When you take a breath, where do you turn your head to look at the victim?

6. While blowing into the victim's nose, what do you do with the person's mouth?

7. In which position is the airway of an unconscious person less likely to be blocked by fluids such as blood and vomit?

8. What is the first step in finding where to give chest compressions?

9. How far do you compress the chest of an adult?

10. At what rate do you give chest compressions to an adult in one-rescuer CPR?

11. How do you count for a rate of 80 compressions per minute?

12. In one-rescuer CPR, what is the pattern of compressions and breaths?

13. When compressing the chest, how do you keep your elbows?

14. What kind of surface should the victim be on when receiving CPR?

15. What should you do if a person coughs forcefully but appears to be choking?

16. When you give abdominal thrusts, what part of your fist do you place against the victim?

17. When giving abdominal thrusts to a woman whose airway is completely blocked and she begins to cough forcefully, what should you do?

18. What should you do when giving abdominal thrusts to a choking victim who loses consciousness?

19. When giving breaths to an infant, where should you put your mouth?

20. How big is a slow, gentle breath for an infant or baby?

21. When you administer back blows to an infant or baby, where should the victim's head be?

22. Where do you check the pulse of an infant or baby?

23. Where do you push on the chest of an infant or baby?

24. How far do you compress the chest of an infant or baby?

25. Where do you push on the chest of a child?

Surgical and Advanced Intervention for the Cardiac Patient

14

TERMINAL OBJECTIVE

To provide the student with a brief overview and understanding of some of the more frequently used modes of surgical and advanced intervention for the cardiac patient.

COMPETENCY OBJECTIVES

Upon completion of this chapter, the student will be able to

1. Describe when it may be necessary to perform a more advanced intervention or surgery on a cardiac patient.
2. Discuss the purpose of testing for central venous pressure.
3. Discuss the purpose and application of a Swan-Ganz catheter.
4. Discuss the purpose of performing a pericardiocentesis.
5. Discuss the purpose of performing a direct current countershock and explain when it is primarily used.
6. Explain the purpose of inserting a cardiac pacemaker and describe the two types most commonly used.
7. Discuss the purpose of performing heart surgery and explain some of the physical and psychosocial considerations involved in caring for the patient who undergoes heart surgery.

While the majority of dysfunctions seen in the heart may be readily diagnosed with the help of the electrocardiogram and X-ray and laboratory studies, some patients may suffer from cardiac problems that require the use of the more advanced and sophisticated types of intervention and surgery currently in use. Some of these procedures include the measurement of central venous pressure, the use of the Swan-Ganz catheter for measuring the pressure in the pulmonary artery, the application of pericardiocentesis, direct current countershock for ventricular fibrillation, and rotating tourniquets.

In addition to the more sophisticated procedures being used to assist physicians in diagnosing disorders affecting the heart, the use of surgical intervention is also a widely accepted method for treating the cardiac patient. Two of the surgeries, the insertion of the electrical pacemaker and the actual surgery upon the heart itself, are presently being performed throughout most of the world.

CENTRAL VENOUS PRESSURE

Central venous pressure, or CVP, is defined as the pressure within the right atrium or in the great veins located within the thorax. Measurement of this pressure helps the physician to determine the need for fluid replacement in a seriously ill patient. It also assists in the evaluation of the pressures in the right atrium and central veins. Finally, it is also used as an aid in diagnosing complete circulatory failure. (See Figure 14–1.)

MEASURING PULMONARY ARTERY PRESSURE

Application of the Swan-Ganz Catheter

Use of the Swan-Ganz catheter helps the physician to monitor the pressure built up in the pulmonary artery. This provides the physician with pertinent information regarding the intravascular filling volume and the cardiac competence of the heart. In addition, it provides a useful assessment of the left heart function, helps to determine cardiac output, and gives a sampling of mixed venous blood.

The purpose of inserting the Swan-Ganz catheter is to obtain measurements in the right atrium, right ventricle, and pulmonary artery, and in the distal branches of the pulmonary artery. It also permits ra-

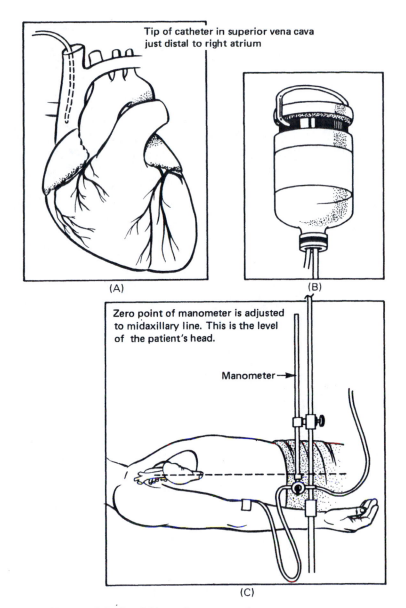

Tip of catheter in superior vena cava just distal to right atrium

(A)

(B)

Zero point of manometer is adjusted to midaxillary line. This is the level of the patient's head.

Manometer →

(C)

Figure 14–1   Measuring central venous pressure.

tional selection of therapy when critical changes may be occurring in the cardiac dynamics, such as in the case of cardiogenic shock, heart failure, and pulmonary edema. (See Figure 14–2.)

PERICARDIOCENTESIS

Pericardiocentesis is the puncturing of the pericardial sac that surrounds the heart in order to aspirate fluid and thereby relieve cardiac tamponade, a condition caused by the compression of the heart by blood, effusion, or a foreign body in the pericardial sac, thus restricting normal heart action.

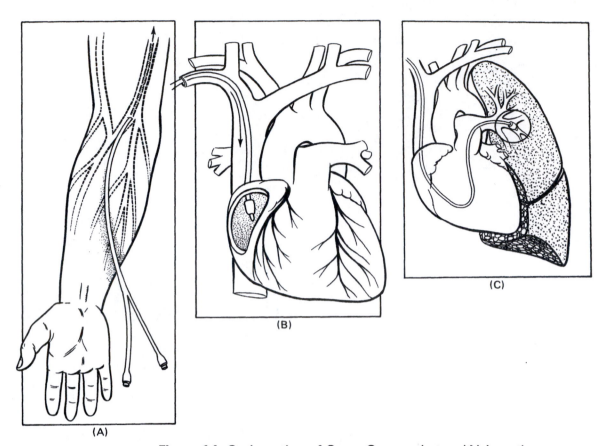

Figure 14–2 Insertion of Swan-Ganz catheter: (A) insertion of catheter into arm; (B) entering the heart; (C) wedged in place in pulmonary artery.

The purpose of performing this procedure is to assist in the removal of fluids from the pericardial sac that may have been caused by pericarditis, or inflammation of the pericardium. In addition to its usefulness in removing the accumulated fluid, this procedure also helps the physician in determining the patient's diagnosis based on the analysis of this fluid. It may also be used as a route of administering certain therapeutic medications. (See Figure 14–3.)

DIRECT CURRENT COUNTERSHOCK USED DURING VENTRICULAR FIBRILLATION

The application of direct current countershock, or electrical discharge, is most useful in terminating ventricular fibrillation. When performed, the use of what is known as a *defibrillator,* applied to the patient's chest, delivers an electric shock that stimulates the heart to convert the ventricular fibrillation to a normal sinus rhythm. (See Figure 14–4.)

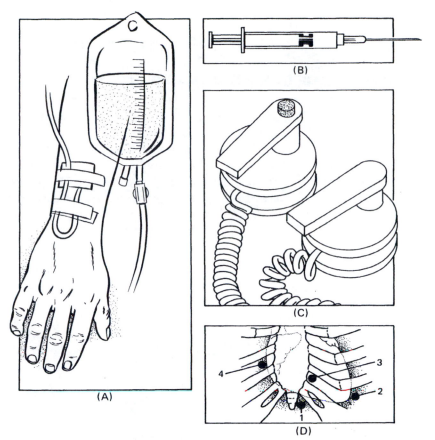

Figure 14–3 Preparing the patient for pericardiocentesis:
(A) intravenous infusion in place; (B) premedication with bar-
bituates for relaxation; (C) emergency equipment ready, if
needed; (D) pericardiocentesis sites.

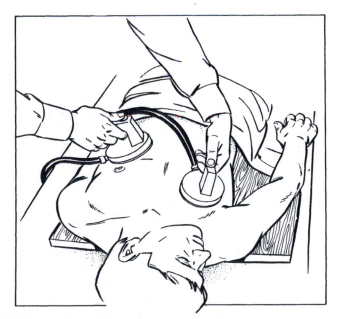

Figure 14–4 Paddle placement for direct current countershock during ventricular fibrillation.

223

APPLICATION OF ROTATING TOURNIQUETS

The use of *rotating tourniquets* refers to a technique whereby tourniquets are systematically rotated on the extremities of the patient in order to remove a volume of blood from the central circulation. In turn, this decreases the venous return and eventually reduces acute pulmonary edema. In addition, it also helps to pool the blood temporarily in the extremities so as to reduce venous return to the heart. (See Figure 14–5.)

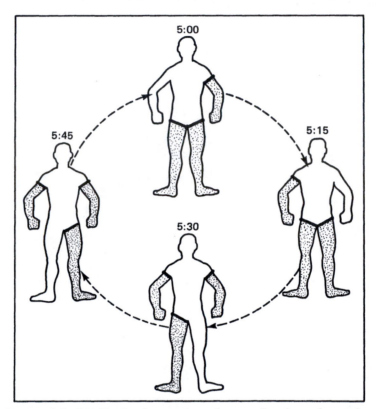

Figure 14–5 Clockwise pattern for application of rotating tourniquets.

INSERTION OF A CARDIAC PACEMAKER

A *pacemaker* is an electronic device that provides repetitive electrical stimuli to the heart muscle for the control of the heart rate. It does this by initiating and maintaining the heart rate when the natural pacemakers of the heart are unable to do so.

The insertion of a cardiac pacemaker is performed as a result of a dysfunction within the heart, as in the cases of heart block, especially those complicated by the Stokes-Adams syndrome, bradycardias and tachycardias, arrhythmias and conduction defects following an acute myocardial infarction, and following open heart surgery and during coronary arteriography. (See Figure 14–6.)

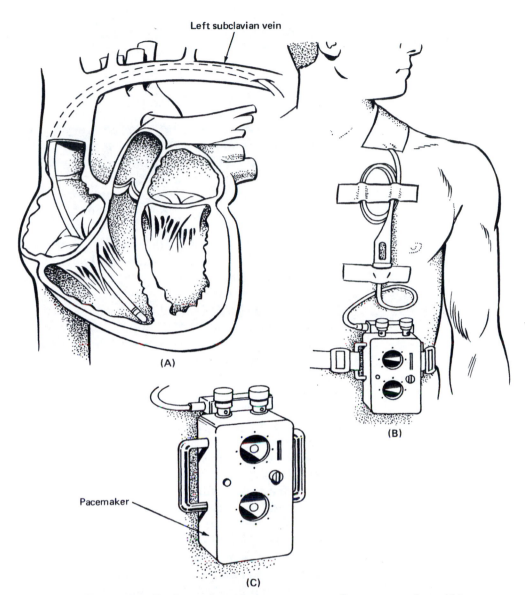

Left subclavian vein

(A)

(B)

Pacemaker

(C)

Figure 14-6 Insertion of temporary cardiac pacemaker: (A)
Insertion of pacemaker line into left subclavian vein; (B) line
in place in heart, attached to outside pacemaker; (C) close
up of outside pacemaker pack.

There are two basic types of cardiac pacemakers that can be inserted
to assist the diseased heart. The first, called a *demand,* or *standby
pacemaker,* is most commonly used. It has the advantage of working only when the heart rate goes below a certain level. Therefore, it does not
compete with the heart's own basic rhythm but, rather, stimulates the
heart when a normal ventricular depolarization does not occur or if the
heart rate drops below a specified rate.

The second type of pacemaker, called a *fixed rate* or *asynchronous
system,* stimulates the ventricle at a preset constant rate that is independ-
ent of the patient's own rhythm. However, it can compete with the pa-

tient's own rhythm, and therefore may be used for patients suffering from either a complete or an unvarying heart block.

HEART SURGERY

The purpose of performing heart surgery is to bring the patient to the peak of his or her physical and psychological capabilities. To do so, however, involves the commitment of all members of the health care team providing care and treatment to the patient.

Surgical intervention of the heart may be performed for a number of reasons, and it may be the treatment of choice for both congenital and acquired diseases affecting both the heart and the great vessels. Some of the more common heart deficiencies that surgery may correct include patent ductus arteriosus, atrial septal defects, tetralogy of Fallot, mitral stenosis, heart block, and coronary artery occlusive disease.

The use of cardiac surgery as a means of correcting the diseased heart involves both physical and psychological intervention. This includes providing the patient with support as he or she undergoes diagnostic studies to determine the type and severity of specific lesions that will need to be operated on. Such support also includes evaluating the patient's emotional state and trying to reduce his or her anxieties before and after the surgery.

The treatment as well as the recovery of the patient undergoing heart surgery will depend extensively upon the reason for performing the surgery and the care provided before, during, and after the operation. This includes not only the emotional and psychological support but also the assessment of specific laboratory studies, the preparation of the patient for events that will occur during the postoperative period, and the use and application of certain drugs and medications that the patient will need before and after surgery. Treatment will also involve many people caring for the patient, such as the nursing staff, members of the respiratory therapy and EKG departments, and X-ray technicians. It is a team effort, and as with the majority of all clinical procedures, it involves a deep commitment from all members of the health care team.

REVIEW QUESTIONS

Directions: For the questions below, give the answers you believe are most correct:

1. _____ _____ _____
   is the pressure within the right atrium or in the great veins located within the thorax.

2. Measuring the _____ _____ _____
   _____ helps the physician to determine the need for fluid replacement in a seriously ill patient.

3. The insertion of a _____ _____
   catheter helps the physician to monitor pressure built up in the _____
   _____ artery.

4. What is the purpose of performing pericardiocentesis?

5. The application of direct current countershock is most useful in terminating

   _____ _____ .

6. When is the application of rotating tourniquets most useful?

7. A _____ is an electronic device that provides repetitive electrical stimuli to the heart muscle in order to control the heart's rate.

8. The purpose of heart surgery is to bring the patient to the peak of his

   _____ and _____ capabilities.

9. Surgical intervention of the heart may be the treatment of choice in both

   _____ and _____ diseases affecting the heart and the great vessels.

10. Who is responsible for providing care and treatment to the heart surgery patient?

EKG Tracings:
Practice Sheets

MEASURING INTERVALS

Directions

For each of the rhythm strips below, measure the PR interval and the QRS complex. As you do each strip, check with the answer key in Appendix B.

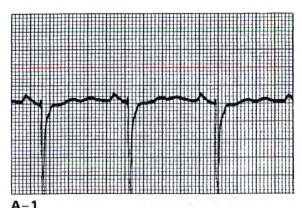

(Reprinted with permission from *Basic Arrhythmias, 3/E* by Gail Walraven, Prentice Hall, Inc., Englewood Cliffs, NJ 07632.)

A–1

PRI: _____ seconds
QRS: _____ seconds

(Reprinted with permission from *Basic Arrhythmias, 3/E* by Gail Walraven, Prentice Hall, Inc., Englewood Cliffs, NJ 07632.)

A–2

PRI: _____ seconds
QRS: _____ seconds

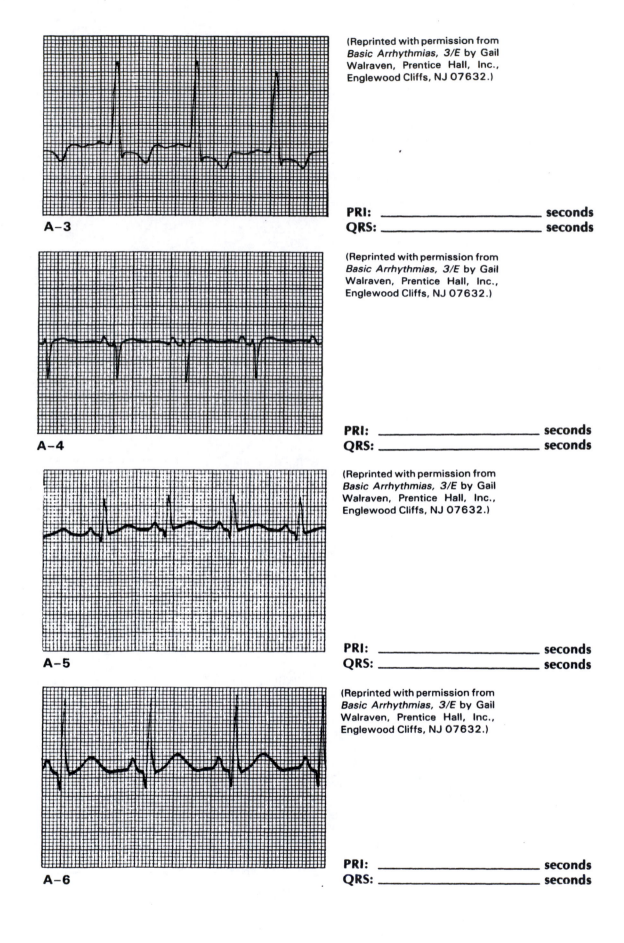

A-3

PRI: _____ seconds
QRS: _____ seconds

A-4

PRI: _____ seconds
QRS: _____ seconds

A-5

PRI: _____ seconds
QRS: _____ seconds

A-6

PRI: _____ seconds
QRS: _____ seconds

ANALYZING EKG STRIPS

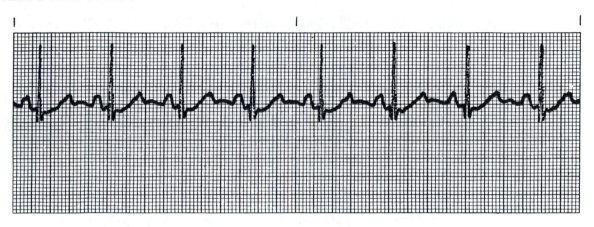

(Reprinted with permission from *Basic Arrhythmias, 3/E* by Gail Walraven,
Prentice Hall, Inc., Englewood Cliffs, NJ 07632.)

A–7   Regularity: _____
           Rate: _____
           P Waves: _____
           PRI: _____
           QRS: _____

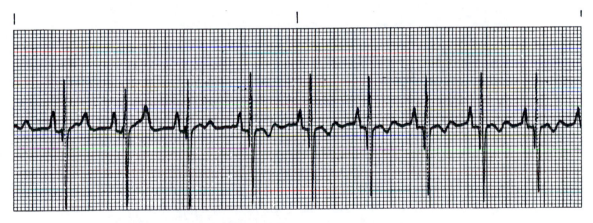

(Reprinted with permission from *Basic Arrhythmias, 3/E* by Gail Walraven,
Prentice Hall, Inc., Englewood Cliffs, NJ 07632.)

A–8   Regularity: _____
           Rate: _____
           P Waves: _____
           PRI: _____
           QRS: _____

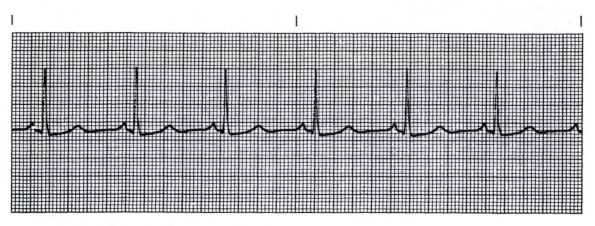

(Reprinted with permission from *Basic Arrhythmias, 3/E* by Gail Walraven,
Prentice Hall, Inc., Englewood Cliffs, NJ 07632.)

A–9   Regularity: _____
                 Rate: _____
                 P Waves: _____
                 PRI: _____
                 QRS: _____

(Reprinted with permission from *Basic Arrhythmias, 3/E* by Gail Walraven,
Prentice Hall, Inc., Englewood Cliffs, NJ 07632.)

A–10   Regularity: _____
                 Rate: _____
                 P Waves: _____
                 PRI: _____
                 QRS: _____

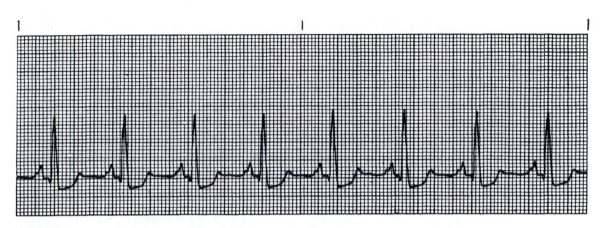

(Reprinted with permission from *Basic Arrhythmias, 3/E* by Gail Walraven,
Prentice Hall, Inc., Englewood Cliffs, NJ 07632.)

A–11   Regularity: _____

Rate: _____

P Waves: _____

PRI: _____

QRS: _____

SINUS RHYTHMS

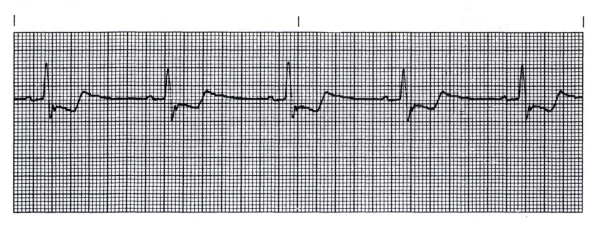

(Reprinted with permission from *Basic Arrhythmias, 3/E* by Gail Walraven,
Prentice Hall, Inc., Englewood Cliffs, NJ 07632.)

A–12   Regularity: _____
              Rate: _____
              P Waves: _____
              PRI: _____
              QRS: _____
              Interp: _____

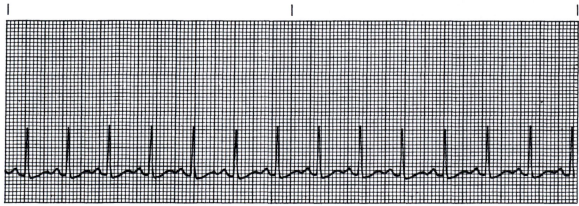

(Reprinted with permission from *Basic Arrhythmias, 3/E* by Gail Walraven,
Prentice Hall, Inc., Englewood Cliffs, NJ 07632.)

A–13   Regularity: _____
              Rate: _____
              P Waves: _____
              PRI: _____
              QRS: _____
              Interp: _____

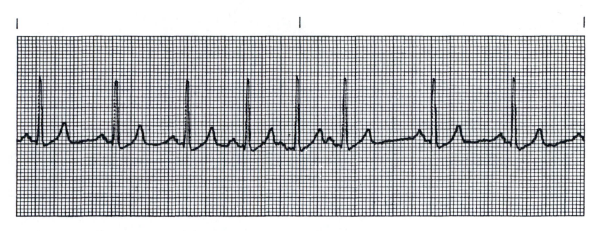

(Reprinted with permission from *Basic Arrhythmias, 3/E* by Gail Walraven, Prentice Hall, Inc., Englewood Cliffs, NJ 07632.)

A-14   Regularity: _____
             Rate: _____
             P Waves: _____
             PRI: _____
             QRS: _____
             Interp: _____

(Reprinted with permission from *Basic Arrhythmias, 3/E* by Gail Walraven, Prentice Hall, Inc., Englewood Cliffs, NJ 07632.)

A-15   Regularity: _____
             Rate: _____
             P Waves: _____
             PRI: _____
             QRS: _____
             Interp: _____

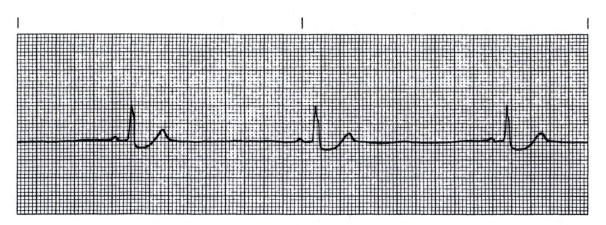

(Reprinted with permission from *Basic Arrhythmias, 3/E* by Gail Walraven,
Prentice Hall, Inc., Englewood Cliffs, NJ 07632.)

A–16   Regularity: _____
             Rate: _____
             P Waves: _____
             PRI: _____
             QRS: _____
             Interp: _____

(Reprinted with permission from *Basic Arrhythmias, 3/E* by Gail Walraven,
Prentice Hall, Inc., Englewood Cliffs, NJ 07632.)

A–17   Regularity: _____
             Rate: _____
             P Waves: _____
             PRI: _____
             QRS: _____
             Interp: _____

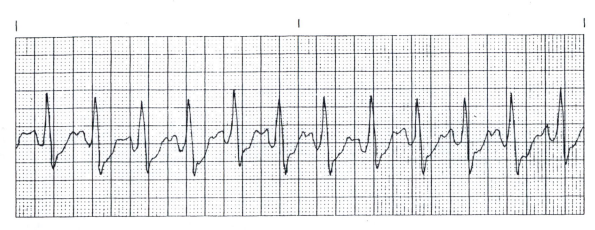

(Reprinted with permission from *Basic Arrhythmias, 3/E* by Gail Walraven, Prentice Hall, Inc., Englewood Cliffs, NJ 07632.)

A-18   Regularity: _____
Rate: _____
P Waves: _____
PRI: _____
QRS: _____
Interp: _____

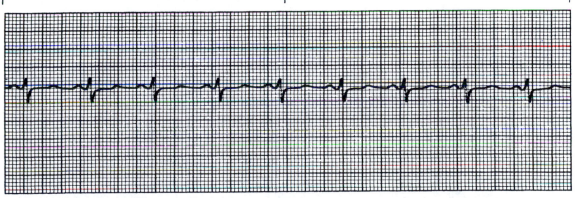

(Reprinted with permission from *Basic Arrhythmias, 3/E* by Gail Walraven, Prentice Hall, Inc., Englewood Cliffs, NJ 07632.)

A-19   Regularity: _____
Rate: _____
P Waves: _____
PRI: _____
QRS: _____
Interp: _____

ATRIAL RHYTHMS

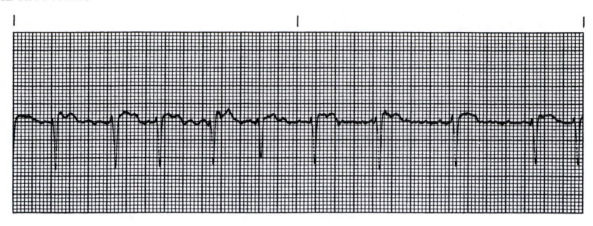

(Reprinted with permission from *Basic Arrhythmias, 3/E* by Gail Walraven,
Prentice Hall, Inc., Englewood Cliffs, NJ 07632.)

A–20   Regularity: _____
             Rate: _____
             P Waves: _____
             PRI: _____
             QRS: _____
             Interp: _____

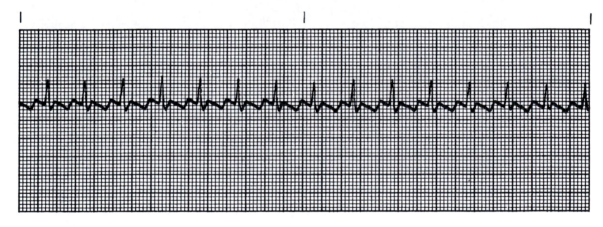

(Reprinted with permission from *Basic Arrhythmias, 3/E* by Gail Walraven,
Prentice Hall, Inc., Englewood Cliffs, NJ 07632.)

A–21   Regularity: _____
             Rate: _____
             P Waves: _____
             PRI: _____
             QRS: _____
             Interp: _____

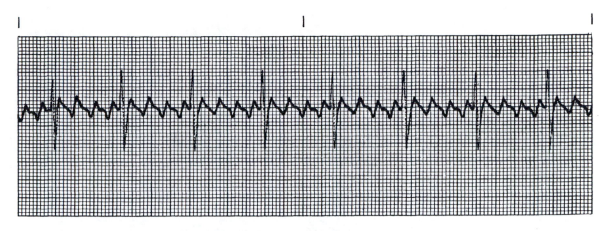

(Reprinted with permission from *Basic Arrhythmias, 3/E* by Gail Walraven,
Prentice Hall, Inc., Englewood Cliffs, NJ 07632.)

A–22

Regularity: _____
Rate: _____
P Waves: _____
PRI: _____
QRS: _____
Interp: _____

(Reprinted with permission from *Basic Arrhythmias, 3/E* by Gail Walraven,
Prentice Hall, Inc., Englewood Cliffs, NJ 07632.)

A–23

Regularity: _____
Rate: _____
P Waves: _____
PRI: _____
QRS: _____
Interp: _____

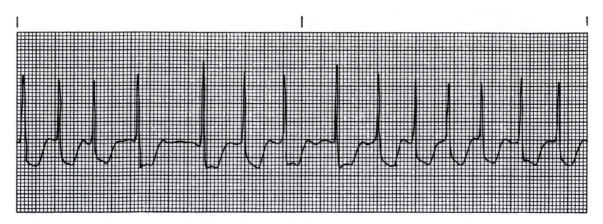

(Reprinted with permission from *Basic Arrhythmias, 3/E* by Gail Walraven,
Prentice Hall, Inc., Englewood Cliffs, NJ 07632.)

A–24   Regularity: _____

Rate: _____

P Waves: _____

PRI: _____

QRS: _____

Interp: _____

(Reprinted with permission from *Basic Arrhythmias, 3/E* by Gail Walraven,
Prentice Hall, Inc., Englewood Cliffs, NJ 07632.)

A–25   Regularity: _____

Rate: _____

P Waves: _____

PRI: _____

QRS: _____

Interp: _____

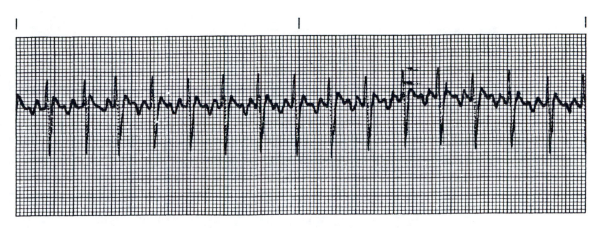

(Reprinted with permission from *Basic Arrhythmias, 3/E* by Gail Walraven, Prentice Hall, Inc., Englewood Cliffs, NJ 07632.)

A-26   Regularity: _____
             Rate: _____
             P Waves: _____
             PRI: _____
             QRS: _____
             Interp: _____

(Reprinted with permission from *Basic Arrhythmias, 3/E* by Gail Walraven, Prentice Hall, Inc., Englewood Cliffs, NJ 07632.)

A-27   Regularity: _____
             Rate: _____
             P Waves: _____
             PRI: _____
             QRS: _____
             Interp: _____

HEART BLOCKS

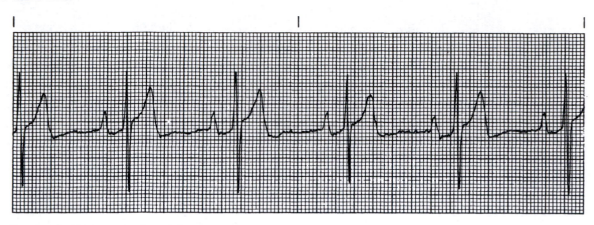

(Reprinted with permission from *Basic Arrhythmias, 3/E* by Gail Walraven,
Prentice Hall, Inc., Englewood Cliffs, NJ 07632.)

A–28   Regularity: _____
             Rate: _____
             P Waves: _____
             PRI: _____
             QRS: _____
             Interp: _____

(Reprinted with permission from *Basic Arrhythmias, 3/E* by Gail Walraven,
Prentice Hall, Inc., Englewood Cliffs, NJ 07632.)

A–29   Regularity: _____
             Rate: _____
             P Waves: _____
             PRI: _____
             QRS: _____
             Interp: _____

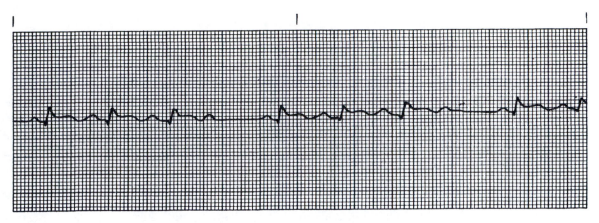

(Reprinted with permission from *Basic Arrhythmias, 3/E* by Gail Walraven, Prentice Hall, Inc., Englewood Cliffs, NJ 07632.)

A–30   Regularity: _____
             Rate: _____
             P Waves: _____
             PRI: _____
             QRS: _____
             Interp: _____

(Reprinted with permission from *Basic Arrhythmias, 3/E* by Gail Walraven, Prentice Hall, Inc., Englewood Cliffs, NJ 07632.)

A–31   Regularity: _____
             Rate: _____
             P Waves: _____
             PRI: _____
             QRS: _____
             Interp: _____

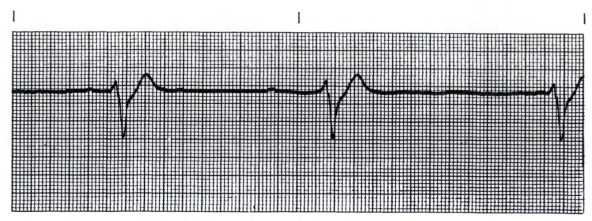

(Reprinted with permission from *Basic Arrhythmias, 3/E* by Gail Walraven,
Prentice Hall, Inc., Englewood Cliffs, NJ 07632.)

A–32   Regularity: _____

Rate: _____

P Waves: _____

PRI: _____

QRS: _____

Interp: _____

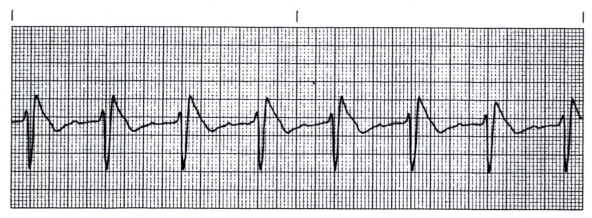

(Reprinted with permission from *Basic Arrhythmias, 3/E* by Gail Walraven,
Prentice Hall, Inc., Englewood Cliffs, NJ 07632.)

A–33   Regularity: _____

Rate: _____

P Waves: _____

PRI: _____

QRS: _____

Interp: _____

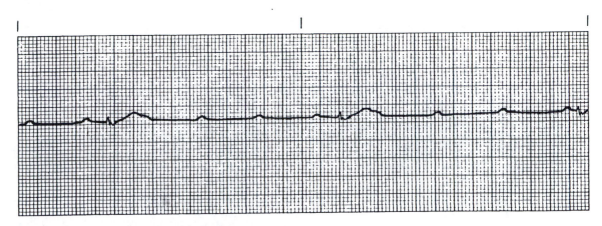

(Reprinted with permission from *Basic Arrhythmias, 3/E* by Gail Walraven,
Prentice Hall, Inc., Englewood Cliffs, NJ 07632.)

A-34   Regularity: _____
       Rate: _____
       P Waves: _____
       PRI: _____
       QRS: _____
       Interp: _____

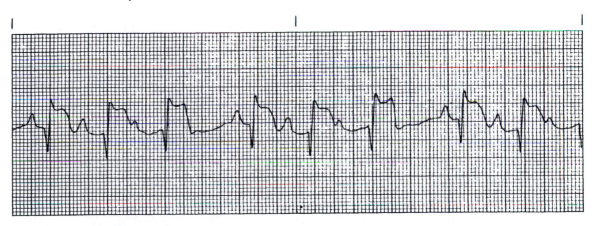

(Reprinted with permission from *Basic Arrhythmias, 3/E* by Gail Walraven,
Prentice Hall, Inc., Englewood Cliffs, NJ 07632.)

A-35   Regularity: _____
       Rate: _____
       P Waves: _____
       PRI: _____
       QRS: _____
       Interp: _____

VENTRICULAR RHYTHMS

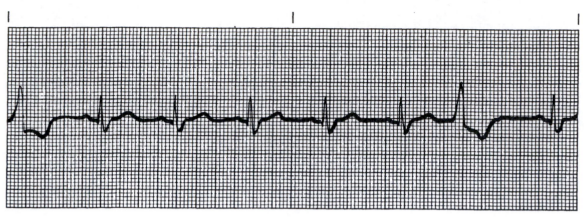

(Reprinted with permission from *Basic Arrhythmias, 3/E* by Gail Walraven,
Prentice Hall, Inc., Englewood Cliffs, NJ 07632.)

A–36   Regularity: _____
       Rate: _____
       P Waves: _____
       PRI: _____
       QRS: _____
       Interp: _____

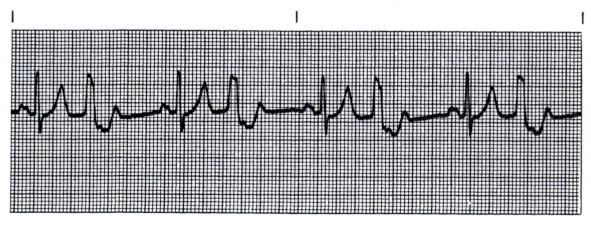

(Reprinted with permission from *Basic Arrhythmias, 3/E* by Gail Walraven,
Prentice Hall, Inc., Englewood Cliffs, NJ 07632.)

A–37   Regularity: _____
       Rate: _____
       P Waves: _____
       PRI: _____
       QRS: _____
       Interp: _____

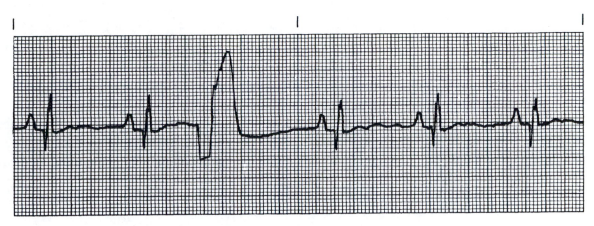

(Reprinted with permission from *Basic Arrhythmias, 3/E* by Gail Walraven,
Prentice Hall, Inc., Englewood Cliffs, NJ 07632.)

A–38   Regularity: _____
             Rate: _____
             P Waves: _____
             PRI: _____
             QRS: _____
             Interp: _____

(Reprinted with permission from *Basic Arrhythmias, 3/E* by Gail Walraven,
Prentice Hall, Inc., Englewood Cliffs, NJ 07632.)

A–39   Regularity: _____
             Rate: _____
             P Waves: _____
             PRI: _____
             QRS: _____
             Interp: _____

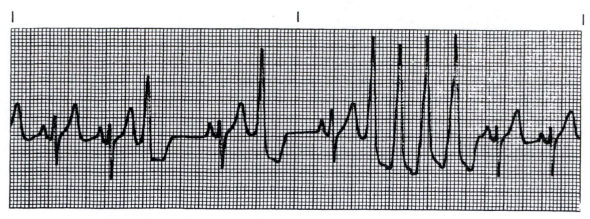

(Reprinted with permission from *Basic Arrhythmias, 3/E* by Gail Walraven,
Prentice Hall, Inc., Englewood Cliffs, NJ 07632.)

A–40   Regularity: _____
             Rate: _____
             P Waves: _____
             PRI: _____
             QRS: _____
             Interp: _____

(Reprinted with permission from *Basic Arrhythmias, 3/E* by Gail Walraven,
Prentice Hall, Inc., Englewood Cliffs, NJ 07632.)

A–41   Regularity: _____
             Rate: _____
             P Waves: _____
             PRI: _____
             QRS: _____
             Interp: _____

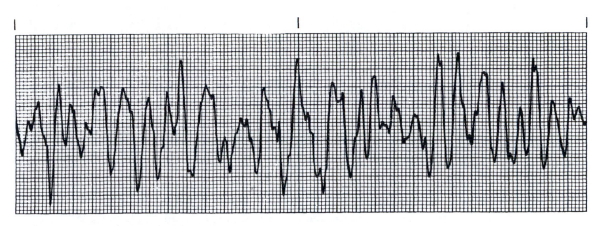

(Reprinted with permission from *Basic Arrhythmias, 3/E* by Gail Walraven,
Prentice Hall, Inc., Englewood Cliffs, NJ 07632.)

A-42   Regularity: _____
             Rate: _____
             P Waves: _____
             PRI: _____
             QRS: _____
             Interp: _____

(Reprinted with permission from *Basic Arrhythmias, 3/E* by Gail Walraven,
Prentice Hall, Inc., Englewood Cliffs, NJ 07632.)

A-43   Regularity: _____
             Rate: _____
             P Waves: _____
             PRI: _____
             QRS: _____
             Interp: _____

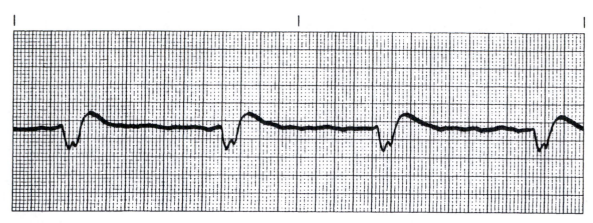

(Reprinted with permission from *Basic Arrhythmias, 3/E* by Gail Walraven,
Prentice Hall, Inc., Englewood Cliffs, NJ 07632.)

A–44   Regularity: _____
                 Rate: _____
                 P Waves: _____
                 PRI: _____
                 QRS: _____
                 Interp: _____

(Reprinted with permission from *Basic Arrhythmias, 3/E* by Gail Walraven,
Prentice Hall, Inc., Englewood Cliffs, NJ 07632.)

A–45   Regularity: _____
                 Rate: _____
                 P Waves: _____
                 PRI: _____
                 QRS: _____
                 Interp: _____

Answers to EKG Tracings: Practice Sheets

B

MEASURING INTERVALS

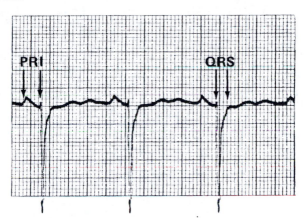

B–1

PRI: .18 seconds
QRS: .12 seconds

(Reprinted with permission from *Basic Arrhythmias, 3/E* by Gail Walraven, Prentice Hall, Inc., Englewood Cliffs, NJ 07632.)

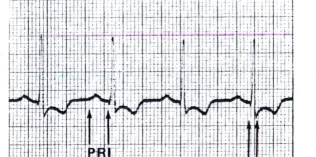

B–2

PRI: .20 seconds
QRS: .08 seconds

(Reprinted with permission from *Basic Arrhythmias, 3/E* by Gail Walraven, Prentice Hall, Inc., Englewood Cliffs, NJ 07632.)

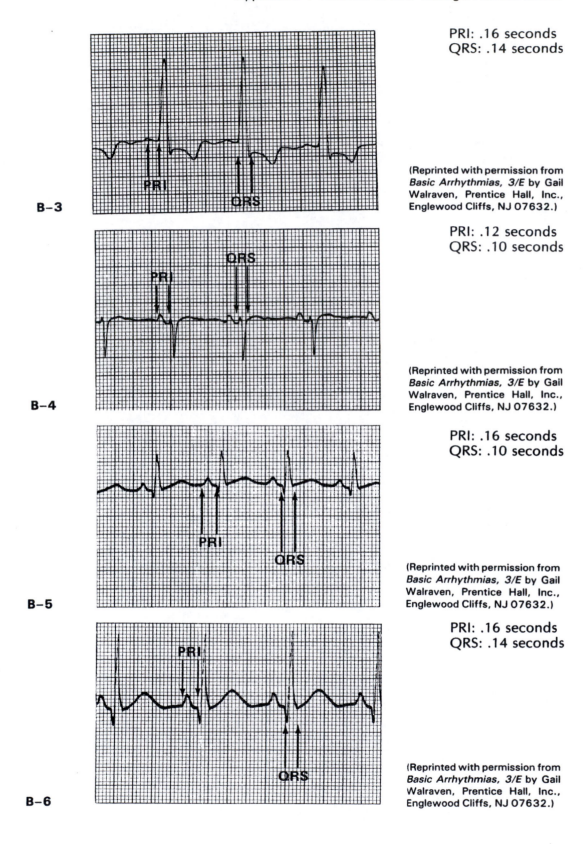

PRI: .16 seconds
QRS: .14 seconds

B-3

PRI: .12 seconds
QRS: .10 seconds

B-4

PRI: .16 seconds
QRS: .10 seconds

B-5

PRI: .16 seconds
QRS: .14 seconds

B-6

ANALYZING EKG STRIPS

B–7	Regularity:	regular
	Rate:	79 beats per minute
	P Waves:	regular P–P interval; uniform waves
	PRI:	.16 seconds and constant
	QRS:	.08 seconds
B–8	Regularity:	irregular
	Rate:	approximately 100 beats per minute
	P Waves:	uniform; regular P–P interval
	PRI:	.12 seconds and constant
	QRS:	.08 seconds
B–9	Regularity:	regular
	Rate:	63 beats per minute
	P Waves:	uniform; regular P–P interval
	PRI:	.16 seconds and constant
	QRS:	.10 seconds
B–10	Regularity:	regular
	Rate:	125 beats per minute
	P Waves:	uniform, regular P–P interval
	PRI:	.16 seconds and constant
	QRS:	.08 seconds
B–11	Regularity:	regular
	Rate:	81 beats per minute
	P Waves:	uniform; regular P–P interval
	PRI:	.16 seconds and constant
	QRS:	.12 seconds

SINUS RHYTHMS

B–12	Regularity:	regular (slightly irregular)
	Rate:	48 beats per minute
	P Waves:	uniform and upright; regular P–P interval
	PRI:	.18 seconds and constant
	QRS:	.12 seconds
	Interp:	Sinus Bradycardia
B–13	Regularity:	regular
	Rate:	136 beats per minute
	P Waves:	uniform and upright; regular P–P interval
	PRI:	.16 seconds and constant
	QRS:	.06 seconds
	Interp:	Sinus Tachycardia

B–14   Regularity: irregular
                 Rate: approximately 80 beats per minute
                 P Waves: uniform P waves with an irregular P–P interval
                 PRI: .16 seconds and constant
                 QRS: .08 seconds
                 Interp: Sinus Arrhythmia

B–15   Regularity: regular
                 Rate: 54 beats per minute
                 P Waves: uniform and upright; regular P–P interval
                 PRI: .16 seconds and constant
                 QRS: .12 seconds
                 Interp: Sinus Bradycardia (with a wide QRS)

B–16   Regularity: slightly irregular
                 Rate: approximately 30 beats per minute
                 P Waves: uniform and upright; irregular P–P interval
                 PRI: .18 seconds and constant
                 QRS: .08 seconds
                 Interp: Sinus Brady-Arrhythmia

B–17   Regularity: irregular
                 Rate: 90 beats per minute
                 P Waves: uniform and upright; irregular P–P interval
                 PRI: .20 seconds and constant
                 QRS: .06 seconds
                 Interp: Sinus Arrhythmia

B–18   Regularity: regular
                 Rate: 115 beats per minute
                 P Waves: uniform and upright; regular P–P interval
                 PRI: .14 seconds and constant
                 QRS: .16 seconds
                 Interp: Sinus Tachycardia

B–19   Regularity: regular
                 Rate: 88 beats per minute
                 P Waves: uniform and upright; regular P–P interval
                 PRI: .16 seconds and constant
                 QRS: .08 seconds
                 Interp: Normal Sinus Rhythm

(Reprinted with permission from *Basic Arrhythmias, 3/E* by Gail Walraven,
Prentice Hall, Inc., Englewood Cliffs, NJ 07632.)

ATRIAL RHYTHMS

B-20
Regularity:	irregular
Rate:	approximately 100 beats per minute
P Waves:	not discernible; only undulations are present
PRI:	none
QRS:	.08 seconds
Interp:	uncontrolled Atrial Fibrillation

B-21
Regularity:	regular
Rate:	atrial rate is 300 beats per minute; ventricular rate is 150 beats per minute
P Waves:	uniform; sawtooth appearance
PRI:	none
QRS:	.10 seconds (QRS is difficult to measure due to obscuring by flutter waves)
Interp:	Atrial Flutter with 2:1 response

B-22
Regularity:	regular
Rate:	atrial rate is 328 beats per minute; ventricular rate is 82 beats per minute
P Waves:	uniform; sawtooth appearance
PRI:	none
QRS:	.08 seconds
Interp:	Atrial Flutter with 4:1 response

B-23
Regularity:	irregular
Rate:	approximately 50 beats per minute
P Waves:	not discernible; undulations present
PRI:	none
QRS:	.08 seconds (QRS complexes are sometimes obscured by fibrillatory waves)
Interp:	controlled Atrial Fibrillation

B-24
Regularity:	irregular
Rate:	approximately 140 beats per minute
P Waves:	not discernible
PRI:	none
QRS:	.06 seconds
Interp:	uncontrolled Atrial Fibrillation

B-25
Regularity:	irregular
Rate:	atrial rate 300 beats per minute; ventricular rate approximately 130 beats per minute
P Waves:	uniform; sawtooth appearance
PRI:	none
QRS:	.08 seconds
Interp:	Atrial Flutter with variable response

(Reprinted with permission from *Basic Arrhythmias, 3/E* by Gail Walraven, Prentice Hall, Inc., Englewood Cliffs, NJ 07632.)

HEART BLOCKS

B–26 Regularity: regular
Rate: atrial rate is 334 beats per minute; ventricular rate is 166 beats per minute
P Waves: uniform; sawtooth appearance; two P waves for every QRS complex
PRI: none
QRS: .10 seconds; slightly obscured by flutter waves
Interp: Atrial Flutter with 2:1 response

B–27 Regularity: irregular
Rate: approximately 40 beats per minute
P Waves: shapes change; P–P interval is irregular
PRI: varies (.12–.16 seconds)
QRS: .08 seconds
Interp: Wandering Pacemaker

B–28 Regularity: regular
Rate: 51 beats per minute
P Waves: uniform and upright; regular P–P interval
PRI: .24 seconds and constant
QRS: .10 seconds
Interp: Sinus Bradycardia with First Degree Heart Block

B–29 Regularity: regular
Rate: 73 beats per minute
P Waves: non-conducted P waves are more apparent after mapping the P–P interval, since some P waves are hidden within the QRS complexes and T waves
PRI: P waves are not associated with QRS complexes
QRS: .08 seconds
Interp: Third Degree Heart Block (CHB) with junctional escape focus

B–30 Regularity: irregular with a pattern of grouped beating
Rate: atrial rate 100 beats per minute; ventricular rate 80 beats per minute
P Waves: uniform; regular P–P interval
PRI: changing; progressively lengthen from .16 seconds to .24 seconds
QRS: .08 seconds
Interp: Wenckebach (Second Degree Heart Block Mobitz I)

B–31 Regularity: regular
Rate: atrial rate 120 beats per minute; ventricular rate 60 beats per minute
P Waves: uniform and upright; regular P–P interval; consistently two P waves for every QRS complex
PRI: .38 seconds and constant
QRS: .10 seconds
Interp: Classical Second Degree Heart Block (Mobitz II) with 2:1 conduction

(Reprinted with permission from *Basic Arrhythmias, 3/E* by Gail Walraven,
Prentice Hall, Inc., Englewood Cliffs, NJ 07632.)

B–32   Regularity: irregular (see note)
                  Rate: approximately 25 beats per minute
                  P Waves: uniform; regular P–P intervals; more P waves than QRS
                              complexes
                  PRI: the P waves are not associated to the QRS complexes
                  QRS: .20 seconds
                  Interp: Third Degree Heart Block (CHB) with ventricular
                              escape focus.
                  Note: The ventricular pacemaker site usually has a regular
                              firing mechanism; but if a dangerous ventricular
                              rhythm is allowed to continue untreated, its serious
                              effects on the myocardium will ultimately cause the
                              firing site to slow or die out. In this strip, the change
                              in ventricular rate demonstrates this slowing
                              phenomenon.

B–33   Regularity: regular
                  Rate: 75 beats per minute
                  P Waves: uniform; regular P–P interval
                  PRI: .30 seconds and constant
                  QRS: .14 seconds
                  Interp: Sinus Rhythm with First Degree Heart Block (with wide
                              QRS)

B–34   Regularity: regular
                  Rate: atrial rate 100 beats per minute; ventricular rate 24
                              beats per minute
                  P Waves: uniform; regular P–P interval; more P waves than QRS
                              complexes
                  PRI: the P waves are not associated with the QRS complexes
                  QRS: .08 seconds
                  Interp: Third Degree Heart Block (CHB) with a junctional es-
                              cape focus
                  Note: The ventricular rate in this strip is slower than the usual
                              junctional rate, but the QRS measurement of .10 sec-
                              onds could not have been produced by a ventricular
                              pacemaker; thus, the escape focus must have been
                              junctional.

B–35   Regularity: irregular with a pattern of grouped beating
                  Rate: atrial rate 107 beats per minute; ventricular rate ap-
                              proximately 90 beats per minute
                  P Waves: uniform; regular P–P interval; more P waves than QRS
                              complexes
                  PRI: changes; progressively lengthens from .20 seconds to
                              .36 seconds
                  QRS: .10 seconds
                  Interp: Wenckebach (Second Degree Heart Block Mobitz I)

(Reprinted with permission from *Basic Arrhythmias*, *3/E* by Gail Walraven,
Prentice Hall, Inc., Englewood Cliffs, NJ 07632.)

VENTRICULAR RHYTHMS

B-36   Regularity: regular underlying rhythm interrupted by ectopics
Rate: 75 beats per minute
P Waves: uniform; regular P–P interval
PRI: .18 seconds
QRS: .12 seconds in underlying complex:
            .12 seconds in ectopics
            ectopics have bizarre configuration
Interp: Sinus Rhythm (with wide QRS) with two PVCs

B-37   Regularity: regular underlying rhythm interrupted by ectopics in a
            pattern of grouped beating
Rate: 39 beats per minute according to visible P waves; true
            sinus rate is probably 78 beats per minute
P Waves: uniform; regular P–P interval
PRI: .18 seconds
QRS: .08 seconds in underlying rhythm: .14 seconds in ectopic
Interp: Sinus Rhythm with bigeminy of PVCs

B-38   Regularity: regular underlying rhythm interrupted by an ectopic
Rate: 60 beats per minute
P Waves: uniform; regular P–P interval
PRI: .20 seconds
QRS: .10 seconds in underlying rhythm;
            .18 seconds in ectopic;
            ectopic has bizarre configuration
Interp: Sinus Rhythm (borderline bradycardia) with one PVC

B-39   Regularity: slightly irregular
Rate: approximately 170 beats per minute
P Waves: not visible
PRI: none
QRS: .12 seconds; configuration is bizarre
Interp: Ventricular Tachycardia

B-40   Regularity: regular underlying rhythm interrupted by ectopics
Rate: 107 beats per minute (underlying rhythm)
P Waves: uniform; regular P–P interval interrupted by ectopics
PRI: .14 seconds
QRS: .10 seconds in underlying rhythm;
            .14 seconds in ectopics;
            ectopics have bizarre configuration
Interp: Sinus Rhythm with two unifocal PVCs and a short burst
            of Ventricular Tachycardia

B-41   Regularity: regular
Rate: 167 beats per minute
P Waves: not visible
PRI: none
QRS: .16 seconds; bizarre configuration
Interp: Ventricular Tachycardia

B–42	Regularity:	totally chaotic baseline
	Rate:	cannot be determined
	P Waves:	none
	PRI:	none
	QRS:	none
	Interp:	Ventricular Fibrillation

B–43	Regularity:	totally chaotic baseline
	Rate:	cannot be determined
	P Waves:	none
	PRI:	none
	QRS:	none
	Interp:	Ventricular Fibrillation

B–44	Regularity:	regular
	Rate:	37 beats per minute
	P Waves:	none
	PRI:	none
	QRS:	.20 seconds; bizarre configuration
	Interp:	Idioventricular Rhythm

B–45	Regularity:	regular underlying rhythm interrupted by ectopics
	Rate:	94 beats per minute (underlying rhythm)
	P Waves:	uniform; regular P–P interval
	PRI:	.24 seconds and constant
	QRS:	.10 seconds in underlying rhythm; .12–.20 seconds in ectopics; ectopics occur consecutively; ectopics have bizarre configuration
	Interp:	Sinus Rhythm with First Degree Heart Block, with one PVC and run of PVCs

(Reprinted with permission from *Basic Arrhythmias, 3/E* by Gail Walraven, Prentice Hall, Inc., Englewood Cliffs, NJ 07632.)

Answers to Review Questions

C

CHAPTER 1

1. William Einthoven
2. To help the physician in diagnosing any irregularities or changes in the patient's heart action
3. Cardiovascular technician; cardiologist; EKG technician I; EKG technician II
4. Treadmill technician; holter recorder scanning technician; echocardiograph technician; cardiac catheterization technician
5. Operate the EKG machine; cut and mount EKG strips; maintain EKG equipment; forward charges for services to billing department; prepare copies of EKG strips; order supplies; notify supervisor immediately of deviations from normal EKG reading.
6. (a) Ability to communicate; (b) coordination of hand and eye movements; (c) enjoys working with people; (d) is interested in both technical and scientific information; (e) works well under pressure
7. Acute-care hospital; medical center; skilled nursing facility; outpatient center; urgent-care facility; private physician's office
8. Vocational

CHAPTER 2

1.
    5   angina pectoris
    7   circulatory
   10   thrombosis
    6   cardiac cycle
    4   hypertension
   19   palpitation
   16   infarct
   12   arrhythmia
    9   stasis
   14   insufficiency
   20   tachycardia

   13   cerebrovascular accident
   21   paroxysmal tachycardia
   11   symptom
   15   bradycardia
    3   pulse
   18   syncope
    1   anoxia
    2   cardiac output

2. | | | | |
    |---|---|---|---|
    | E | QID | G | < |
    | P | QH | D | TPR |
    | B | Stat | H | TID |
    | A | c̄ | L | QD |
    | N | BID | M | s̄ |
    | I | DC | F | SOB |
    | K | p̄ | O | BP |
    | C | > | J | CVA |

3. **(a)** operating room; **(b)** intensive care unit; **(c)** coronary care unit; **(d)** emergency room; **(e)** central supply; **(f)** pediatrics; **(g)** obstetrics; **(h)** laboratory; **(i)** outpatient department; **(j)** eye, ear, nose, and throat

4. **(a)** drop; **(b)** nothing by mouth; **(c)** at liberty; **(d)** whenever necessary; **(e)** quantity sufficient; **(f)** activities of daily living; **(g)** oxygen; **(h)** specimen; **(i)** treatment; **(j)** diagnosis

5. **(a)** 6; **(b)** 7; **(c)** 8; **(d)** 9; **(e)** 10; **(f)** 300; **(g)** 1000; **(h)** 35; **(i)** 19; **(j)** 125

6. **(a)** Joint; **(b)** vessel; **(c)** one, self; **(d)** toward; **(e)** against; **(f)** before; **(g)** heart; **(h)** blood; **(j)** beside; **(i)** within

7. **(a)** Pain; **(b)** recording; **(c)** inflammation; **(d)** bleeding; **(e)** abnormal enlargement; **(f)** discharge; **(g)** repair; **(h)** enlargement; **(i)** to make a surgical opening; **(j)** condition of

8. **(a)** Before meals; **(b)** aqueous (water); **(c)** gram; **(d)** grain; **(e)** hour of sleep; **(f)** intramuscular; **(g)** liter; **(h)** right eye; **(i)** milligram; **(j)** iron

CHAPTER 3

1. Prevent blood from backing up
2. Four
3. To pump blood
4. Aorta
5. Pericardium
6. Lub: closing of the tricuspid and mitral valves; dub: closing of the aortic and pulmonary valves
7. Right atrium; right ventricle
8. Mitral; tricuspid
9. Semilunar
10. Blood enters from the right atrium, then moves through the tricuspid valve to the right ventricle, through the pulmonary semilunar valve, into the lungs, back through the left atrium. Once the blood leaves the left atrium, it flows through the bicuspid, or mitral valve, into the left ventricle, through the aortic semilunar valve, and eventually out to the rest of the body.
11. **(a)** Endocardim (inner layer); **(b)** myocardium (middle layer); **(c)** epicardium (outer layer)
12. Oxygenated; away
13. Deoxygenated; toward
14. Capillaries
15. Lymphatic; thoracic
16. Coronary circulation
17. Depolarization

18. Increases
19. 60; 100
20. (a) Pertains to the time spent during the heart's contraction and relaxation; (b) time in which myocardium completes its contraction; (c) time in which myocardium begins to relax

CHAPTER 4

1. A two-way process, in which information, facts, or feelings may be shared with others.
2. Observation
3. (a) Verbal (oral); (b) written; (c) nonverbal
4. Sender; receiver
5. Care plans; patient's chart
6. Nonverbal
7. Professionalism
8. Nursing; admitting; radiology; cardiopulmonary; EKG department; laboratory
9. Safety; comfort
10. Keeping that which is heard or seen in the hospital confidential
11. Standards and principles inherent to the science and art of medicine
12. Negligence
13. Malpractice
14. Honesty; dependability; integrity
15. (a) Use of drugs or alcohol; (b) patient harm or abuse

CHAPTER 5

1. (a) Standard 12-lead EKG machine; (b) 3-channel computerized EKG machine
2. (a) Electrodes; (b) leads; (c) amplifier; (d) galvanometer; (e) stylus
3. Patient wires
4. Correct attachment of electrodes and leads
5. (a) 4. white; (b) 3. green; (c) 2. black; (d) 1. red
6. (a) Fourth intercostal space, right sternal border; (b) fourth intercostal space, left sternal border; (c) equal distance between V2 and V4; (d) fifth intercostal space, left midclavicular line; (e) lateral, to the side of V4, at the anterior to the mid-axillary line; (f) lateral to V5, at the mid-axillary line
7. (a) Indicates if the machine is ON or OFF; (b) allows the technician to standardize the machine; (c) used to adjust the stylus temperature; (d) used to move the recording up and down on the paper
8. Sensitivity
9. The speed (25 or 50mm/sec) at which the paper drive causes the EKG paper to move
10. Patient cable
11. 25; 1mm; 1mm

12. Heat; pressure
13. Electrolyte
14. Electrolyte; drift

CHAPTER 6

1. Warmth; sleep; food; water; oxygen; elimination; activity
2. (a) Love; (b) understanding
3. The need to communicate
4. Recognize; likes; dislikes
5. (a) Pain; (b) death
6. Spiritual
7. Basic
8. Privacy
9. February 6, 1973
10. 12

CHAPTER 7

1. To record the electrical impulses of the heart, as the blood is pumped through the body
2. Diagnostic tool
3. 40
4. After a myocardial infarction; pre or post surgery; patients with a history of heart disease; routine checkup; if the patient is taking cardiac medications
5. The steps taken in order to ensure the proper operation of the EKG machine and patient preparation for the EKG
6. 12
7. Six
8. Date; time
9. (a) AC interference; (b) somatic tremors; (c) baseline shift; (d) loose or broken wires
10. The computerized machine makes the recording of the EKG easier.
11. History

CHAPTER 8

1. Four
2. Rate; rhythm; conduction; configuration
3. Contraction of the atrial
4. How long it has taken the electrical impulse to travel from the SA node to the bundle of His.
5. The spread of the impulse through the ventricular muscle "depolarization"
6. The resting period between depolarization and repolarization

7. The recovery period of the ventricles

8. Following the T-wave; usually seen in a patient with a potassium deficiency

9. 60–100

10. Abnormally slow heart beat

11. Abnormally fast heart beat

12. Any abnormal heart beat

13. A momentary stopping of the impulse occuring from the SA node.

14. Paroxysmal atrial tachycardia; atrial flutter; atrial fibrillation

15. Ectopic focus; portrayed with an abnormal P-wave configuration, such as flat, slurred, notched, inverted, or wide

16. Premature ventricular contraction

17. Created by stimuli from many ventricular ectopic foci, causing a chaotic twitching of the ventricles

18. By a wide QRS-complex and a regular rhythm

19. Ventriclar standstill; absence of contractions; viewed as a "straight line"

20.

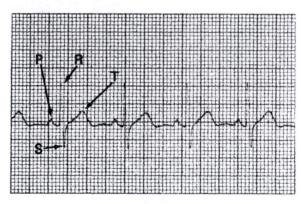

21.

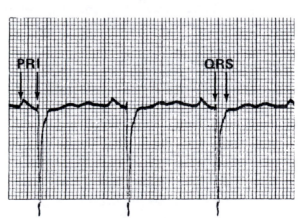

22.

Regularity: irregular
Rate: approximately 100 beats per minute
P Waves: not discernible; only undulations are present
PRI: none
QRS: .08 seconds
Interp: uncontrolled Atrial Filbrillation

23.

Regularity:	regular underlying rhythm interrupted by ectopics
Rate:	75 beats per minute
P Waves:	uniform; regular P-P interval
PRI:	.18 seconds
QRS:	.12 seconds in underlying complex:
	.12 seconds in ectopics
	ectopics have bizarre configuration
Interp:	Sinus Rhythm (with wide QRS) with two PVCs

24.

Regularity:	regular
Rate:	51 beats per minute
P Waves:	uniform and upright; regular P-P interval
PRI:	.24 seconds and constant
QRS:	.10 seconds
Interp:	Sinus Bradycardia with First Degree Heart Block

25.

Regularity:	regular (slightly irregular)
Rate:	48 beats per minute
P Waves:	uniform and upright; regular P-P interval
QRS:	.12 seconds
Interp:	Sinus Bradycardia

CHAPTER 9

1. Diseases affecting the heart and cardiovascular system
2. 55%
3. (a) Dyspnea; (b) chest pain; (c) edema; (d) palpitations; (e) hemoptysis
4. Patent ductus arteriosus; tetralogy of Fallot
5. An inflammation within the external lining of the valves
6. Associated with myocardial infarction, neoplasm, or trauma to the heart
7. Arteriosclerosis; the interior walls of the arteries are subject to a buildup of hardened materials
8. One or more coronary arteries becoming occluded
9. The heart is no longer able to meet the body's demands.
10. (a) Coldness; (b) pallor; (c) rubor; (d) pain; (e) cyanosis
11. There is an enlargement and twisting of superficial veins.
12. Local dilations of blood vessels that bulge out from the vessel walls
13. High blood pressure
14. Coronary heart disease; arteriosclerosis; myocardial infarction; angina; atherosclerosis
15. Rheumatic heart disease; endocarditis; polymyositis

CHAPTER 10

1. The degree of body heat that is a direct result of the balance maintained between heat produced and heat lost by the body
2. Early morning; evening
3. Oral, axillary, rectal; least accurate is axillary; most accurate is rectal
4. The beat of the heart as felt through the walls of the arteries
5. Radial artery
6. Stethoscope
7. Rate; depth; rhythm
8. Age; activity; disease; smoking
9. The pressure of the force of blood against the walls of the arteries, which is measured when the heart contracts and relaxes.
10. Systolic; diastolic
11. 140mmHG
12. 90mmHg
13. Thumb
14. 120/80
15. Sphygmomanometer

CHAPTER 11

1. Heart disease
2. (a) Auscultation; (b) cardiographic studies; (c) roentgenological studies
3. Auscultation
4. Ambulatory electrocardiographic monitoring
5. Ballistocardiogram
6. Phonocardiogram
7. Vectorcardiography
8. Echocardiography
9. Chest x-ray
10. Angiocardiography
11. Cardiac catheterization

CHAPTER 12

1. Cardiac glycosides
2. Digitalis
3. Digoxin; digitoxin
4. Nausea and vomiting; headache; visual disturbances; rashes
5. When arrhythmias develop in the heart
6. Quinidine; procainamide; disopyramide (norpace); lidocaine; phenytocin
7. Propranol
8. Bretylium (Bretyol)
9. Calcium antagonists

10. Verapamil
11. **(a)** Nitrates and nitrites; **(b)** beta-adrenergic blockers; **(c)** calcium antagonists
12. To antagonize or reverse the effects of sympathetic activation caused by exercise and other physical or mental exertions
13. To assist the kidneys in their maintenance of water, electrolytes, and acid-base balance by increasing the amount of urine being produced in the kidneys
14. **(a)** Osmotic; **(b)** thiazide; **(c)** organic acid; **(d)** potassium-sparing
15. Chlorothiazide; hydrochlorothiazide; methyclothiazide; quinethazone
16. Anticoagulants; coagulants

CHAPTER 13

1. **(a)** Determine unresponsiveness; **(b)** call for help; **(c)** open the airway
2. Look at the chest; listen and feel for air coming out of the mouth.
3. three to five seconds
4. In the groove at the side of the neck
5. Chest
6. Close the mouth
7. Lying on the side
8. Trace the lower edge of the rib cage to the notch where the ribs meet the sternum.
9. $1\frac{1}{2}$ to 2 inches
10. 80 to 100 per minute
11. "One-and, two-and, three-and. . ."
12. 15 compressions, then 2 breaths
13. Straight
14. Hard
15. Let him alone and watch.
16. The thumb side
17. Stop right away.
18. Sweep the mouth and attempt to ventilate.
19. Over the baby's mouth and nose
20. Enough air to make the chest rise and fall
21. Lower than the chest
22. In the middle of the upper arm
23. One finger-width below the imaginary nipple line
24. $\frac{1}{2}$ to 1 inch
25. One finger-width up from the sternal notch

CHAPTER 14

1. Central venous pressure
2. Central venous pressure
3. Swan-Ganz

4. Aspirate fluid, in order to relieve cardiac tamponade
5. Ventricular fibrillation
6. In removing volumes of blood in central circulation; reduces acute pulmonary edema
7. Pacemaker
8. Physical; psychological
9. Congenital; acquired
10. All members of the health care team

Index

Flash Cards

D

Electrical Conduction through the Heart

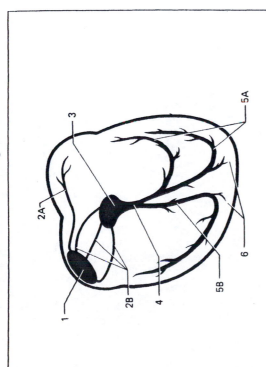

1. Sinoatrial (SA) node
2A. Intraatrial pathway
2B. Internodal pathways
3. Atrioventricular (AV) junction
4. Bundle of His
5A. Left bundle branches (2 divisions)
5B. Right bundle branch
6. Purkinje fibers

Inherent Rates

The inherent rate ranges of the major sites are

SA Node	60–100 beats per minute
AV Junction	40–60 beats per minute
Ventricle	20–40 beats per minute

(Reprinted with permission from *Basic Arrhythmias, 3/E* by Gail Walraven, Prentice Hall, Inc., Englewood Cliffs, NJ 07632.)

(Reprinted with permission from *Basic Arrhythmias, 3/E* by Gail Walraven, Prentice Hall, Inc., Englewood Cliffs, NJ 07632.)

EKG Wave Patterns

Electrical Activity	Associated Pattern	Graphic Depiction
Atrial Depolarization	P Wave	
Delay at AV Node	PR Segment	
Ventricular Depolarization	QRS Complex	
Ventricular Repolarization	T Wave	
No Electrical Activity	Isolectric Line	

(Reprinted with permission from *Basic Arrhythmias, 3/E* by Gail Walraven, Prentice Hall, Inc., Englewood Cliffs, NJ 07632.)

Rate Calculation

METHOD	DIRECTIONS	FEATURES
A	Count the number of R waves in a 6-second strip and multiply by 10.	• not very accurate • used only with very quick estimate
B	Count the number of large squares between 2 consecutive R waves and divide into 300. –OR– *Memorize this Scale:* 1 large square = 300 bpm 2 " " = 150 " 3 " " = 100 " 4 " " = 75 " 5 " " = 60 " 6 " " = 50 "	• very quick • not very accurate with fast rates • only used with regular rhythms
C	Count the number of small squares between 2 consecutive R waves and divide into 1500.	• most accurate • used only with regular rhythms • time consuming

(Reprinted with permission from *Basic Arrhythmias, 3/E* by Gail Walraven, Prentice Hall, Inc., Englewood Cliffs, NJ 07632.)

EKG Complex

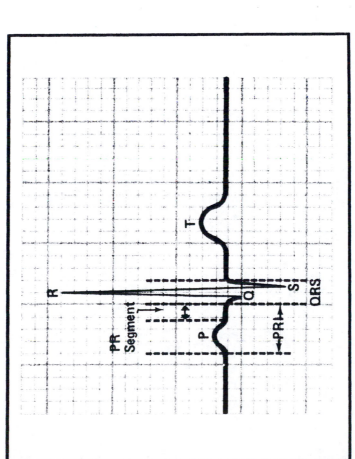

Normal EKG Measurements

PRI: .12–.20 seconds
QRS: < .12 seconds

(Reprinted with permission from *Basic Arrhythmias, 3/E* by Gail Walraven, Prentice Hall, Inc., Englewood Cliffs, NJ 07632.)

(Reprinted with permission from *Basic Arrhythmias, 3/E* by Gail Walraven, Prentice Hall, Inc., Englewood Cliffs, NJ 07632.)

Normal Sinus Rhythm

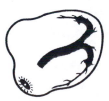

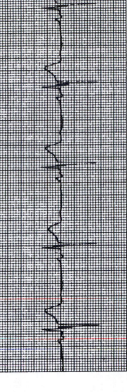

SINUS node is the pacemaker, firing at a regular rate of 60–100 times per minute. Each beat is conducted normally through to the ventricles.

REGULARITY: The R–R intervals are constant; the rhythm is regular.
RATE: The atrial and ventricular rates are equal: heart rate is between 60 and 100 beats per minute.
P WAVE: The P waves are uniform. There is one P wave in front of every QRS complex.
PRI: The PR interval measures between .12 and .20 seconds; the PRI measurement is constant across the strip.
QRS: The QRS complex measures less than .12 seconds.

(Reprinted with permission from *Basic Arrhythmias, 3/E* by Gail Walraven, Prentice Hall, Inc., Englewood Cliffs, NJ 07632.)

Sinus Bradycardia

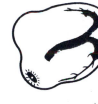

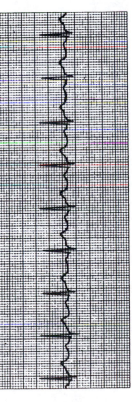

SINUS node is the pacemaker, firing regularly at a rate of less than 60 times per minute. Each impulse is conducted normally through to the ventricles.

REGULARITY: The R–R intervals are constant; the rhythm is regular.
RATE: The atrial and ventricular rates are equal; heart rate is less than 60 beats per minute.
P WAVE: There is a uniform P wave in front of every QRS complex.
PRI: The PR interval measures between .12 and .20 seconds; the PRI measurement is constant across the strip.
QRS: The QRS complex measures less than .12 seconds.

(Reprinted with permission from *Basic Arrhythmias, 3/E* by Gail Walraven, Prentice Hall, Inc., Englewood Cliffs, NJ 07632.)

Sinus Arrhythmia

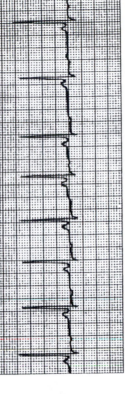

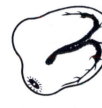

SINUS node is the pacemaker, but impulses are initiated in an irregular pattern. The rate increases as the patient breathes in and decreases as the patient breathes out. Each beat is conducted normally through to the ventricles.

REGULARITY: The R–R intervals vary; the rate changes with the patient's respirations.

RATE: The atrial and ventricular rates are equal; heart rate is usually in a normal range (60–100 beats per minute), but can be slower.

P WAVE: There is a uniform P wave in front of every QRS complex.

PRI: The PR interval measures between .12 and .20 seconds; the PRI measurement is constant across the strip.

QRS: The QRS complex measures less than .12 seconds.

(Reprinted with permission from *Basic Arrhythmias, 3/E* by Gail Walraven. Prentice Hall. Inc.. Englewood Cliffs. NJ 07632.)

Sinus Tachycardia

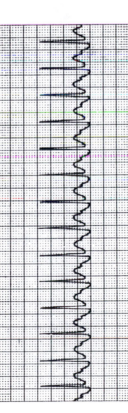

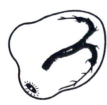

SINUS node is the pacemaker, firing regularly at a rate of greater than 100 times per minute. Each impulse is conducted normally through to the ventricles.

REGULARITY: The R–R intervals are constant; the rhythm is regular.

RATE: The atrial and ventricular rates are equal; the heart rate is greater than 100 beats per minute (usually between 100 and 160 beats per minute).

P WAVE: There is a uniform P wave in front of every QRS complex.

PRI: The PR interval measures between .12 and .20 seconds; the PRI measurement is constant across the strip.

QRS: The QRS complex measures less than .12 seconds.

(Reprinted with permission from *Basic Arrhythmias, 3/E* by Gail Walraven. Prentice Hall. Inc.. Englewood Cliffs. NJ 07632.)

Premature Ventricular Contraction

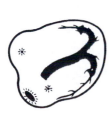

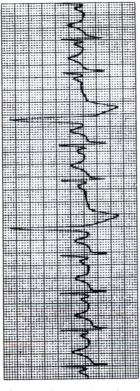

A PVC is a single irritable focus within the VENTRICLES that fires prematurely to initiate an ectopic complex.

REGULARITY: The underlying rhythm can be regular or irregular. The ectopic PVC will interrupt the regularity of the underlying rhythm. PVCs are not usually included in the rate determination because they frequently do not produce a pulse.

RATE: The rate will be determined by the underlying rhythm (unless the PVC is interpolated).

P WAVES: The ectopic is not preceded by a P wave. You may see a coincidental P wave near the PVC, but it is dissociated.

PRI: Since the ectopic comes from a lower focus, there will be no PRI.

QRS: The QRS complex will be wide and bizarre, measuring at least .12 seconds. The configuration will differ from the configuration of the underlying QRS complexes. The T wave is frequently in the opposite direction from the QRS complex.

(Reprinted with permission from *Basic Arrhythmias, 3/E* by Gail Walraven, Prentice Hall, Inc., Englewood Cliffs, NJ 07632.)

Wandering Pacemaker

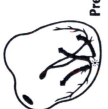

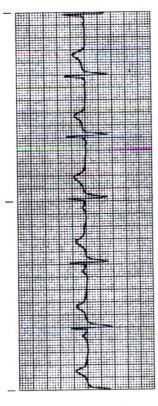

The pacemaker site wanders between the SINUS node, the ATRIA, and the AV JUNCTION. Although each beat originates from a different focus, the rate usually remains within a normal range, but can be slower. Conduction through to the ventricles is normal.

REGULARITY: The R–R intervals vary slightly as the pacemaker site changes; the rhythm can be slightly irregular.

RATE: The atrial and ventricular rates are equal; heart rate is usually within a normal range (60–100 beats per minute) but can be slower.

P WAVE: The morphology of the P wave changes as the pacemaker site changes. There is one P wave in front of every QRS complex, although some may be difficult to see depending on the pacemaker site.

PRI: The PRI measurement will vary slightly as the pacemaker site changes. All PRI measurements should be less than .20 seconds; some may be less than .12 seconds.

QRS: The QRS complex measures less than .12 seconds.

(Reprinted with permission from *Basic Arrhythmias, 3/E* by Gail Walraven, Prentice Hall, Inc., Englewood Cliffs, NJ 07632.)

Atrial Tachycardia

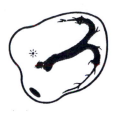

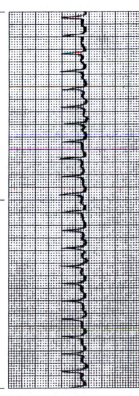

The pacemaker is a single irritable site within the ATRIUM which fires repetitively at a very rapid rate. Conduction through to the ventricles is normal.

REGULARITY: The R–R intervals are constant; the rhythm is regular.

RATE: The atrial and ventricular rates are equal; the heart rate is usually 150–250 beats per minute.

P WAVE: There is one P wave in front of every QRS complex. The configuration of the P wave will be different than that of sinus P waves; they may be flattened or notched. Because of the rapid rate, the P waves can be hidden in the T waves of the preceding beats.

PRI: The PRI is between .12 and .20 seconds and constant across the strip. The PRI may be difficult to measure if the P wave is obscured by the T wave.

QRS: The QRS complex measures less than .12 seconds.

(Reprinted with permission from *Basic Arrhythmias, 3/E* by Gail Walraven, Prentice Hall, Inc., Englewood Cliffs, NJ 07632.)

Atrial Flutter

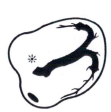

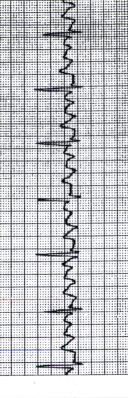

A single irritable focus within the ATRIA issues an impulse that is conducted in a rapid, repetitive fashion. To protect the ventricles from receiving too many impulses, the AV node blocks some of the impulses from being conducted through to the ventricles.

REGULARITY: The atrial rhythm is regular. The ventricular rhythm will be regular if the AV node conducts impulses through in a consistent pattern. If the pattern varies, the ventricular rate will be irregular.

RATE: Atrial rate is between 250 and 350 beats per minute. Ventricular rate will depend on the ratio of impulses conducted through to the ventricles.

P WAVE: When the atria flutter they produce a series of well-defined P waves. When seen together, these "Flutter" waves have a sawtooth appearance.

PRI: Because of the unusual configuration of the P wave (Flutter wave) and the proximity of the wave to the QRS complex, it is often impossible to determine a PRI in this arrhythmia. Therefore, the PRI is not measured in Atrial Flutter.

QRS: The QRS complex measures less than .12 seconds; measurement can be difficult if one or more Flutter waves is concealed within the QRS complex.

(Reprinted with permission from *Basic Arrhythmias, 3/E* by Gail Walraven, Prentice Hall, Inc., Englewood Cliffs, NJ 07632.)

Premature Junctional Contraction

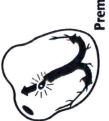

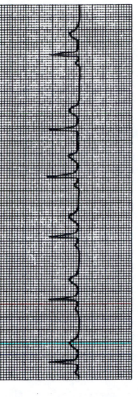

The pacemaker is an irritable focus within the AV JUNCTION which fires prematurely and produces a single ectopic beat. The atria are depolarized via retrograde conduction. Conduction through the ventricles is normal.

REGULARITY: Since this is a single premature ectopic beat, it will interrupt the regularity of the underlying rhythm. The R–R interval will be irregular.

RATE: The overall heart rate will depend on the rate of the underlying rhythm.

P WAVES: The P wave can come before or after the QRS complex, or it can be lost entirely within the QRS complex. If visible, the P wave will be inverted.

PRI: If the P wave precedes the QRS complex, the PRI will be less than .12 seconds. If the P wave falls within the QRS complex or following it, there will be no PRI.

QRS: The QRS complex measurement will be less than .12 seconds.

(Reprinted with permission from *Basic Arrhythmias, 3/E* by Gail Walraven, Prentice Hall, Inc., Englewood Cliffs, NJ 07632.)

Atrial Fibrillation

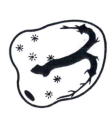

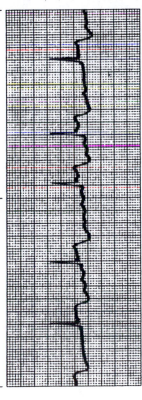

The ATRIA are so irritable that a multitude of foci initiate impulses, causing the atria to depolarize repeatedly in a fibrillatory manner. The AV node blocks most of the impulses, allowing only a limited number through to the ventricles.

REGULARITY: The atrial rhythm is unmeasurable; all atrial activity is chaotic. The ventricular rhythm is grossly irregular having no pattern to its irregularity.

RATE: The atrial rate cannot be measured because it is so chaotic: research indicates that it exceeds 350 beats per minute. The ventricular rate is significantly slower because the AV node blocks most of the impulses. If the ventricular rate is below 100 beats per minute the rhythm is said to be "controlled"; if it is over 100 beats per minute it is considered to have a "rapid ventricular response."

P WAVE: In this arrhythmia the atria are not depolarizing in an effective way; instead, they are fibrillating. Thus, no P wave is produced. All atrial activity is depicted as "fibrillatory" waves, or grossly chaotic undulations of the baseline.

PRI: Since no P waves are visible, no PRI can be measured.

QRS: The QRS complex measurement should be less than .12 seconds.

(Reprinted with permission from *Basic Arrhythmias, 3/E* by Gail Walraven, Prentice Hall, Inc., Englewood Cliffs, NJ 07632.)

Junctional Tachycardia

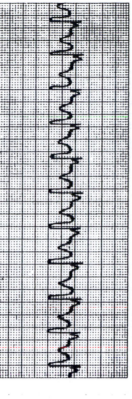

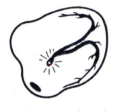

An irritable focus in the AV JUNCTION speeds up to override the SA node for control of the heart. The atria are depolarized via retrograde conduction. Conduction through the ventricles is normal.

REGULARITY: The R–R intervals are constant. The rhythm is regular.
RATE: Atrial and ventricular rates are equal. The rate will be in the tachycardia range, but does not usually exceed 180 beats per minute. Usual range is 100–180 beats per minute.
P WAVES: The P wave can come before or after the QRS complex, or it can be lost entirely within the QRS complex. If visible, the P wave will be inverted.
PRI: If the P wave precedes the QRS complex, the PRI will be less than .12 seconds. If the P wave falls within the QRS complex or following it, there will be no PRI.
QRS: The QRS complex measurement will be less than .12 seconds.

(Reprinted with permission from *Basic Arrhythmias, 3/E* by Gail Walraven, Prentice Hall, Inc., Englewood Cliffs, NJ 07632.)

Junctional Escape Rhythm

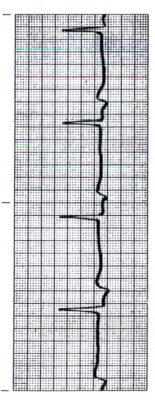

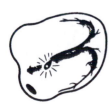

When higher pacemaker sites fail, the AV JUNCTION is left with pacemaking responsibility. The atria are depolarized via retrograde conduction. Ventricular conduction is normal.

REGULARITY: The R–R intervals are constant. The rhythm is regular.
RATE: Atrial and ventricular rates are equal. The inherent rate of the AV Junction is 40–60 beats per minute.
P WAVES: The P wave can come before or after the QRS complex, or it can be lost entirely within the QRS complex. If visible, the P wave will be inverted.
PRI: If the P wave precedes the QRS complex, the PRI will be less than .12 seconds. If the P wave falls within the QRS complex or following it, there will be no PRI.
QRS: The QRS complex measurement will be less than .12 seconds.

(Reprinted with permission from *Basic Arrhythmias, 3/E* by Gail Walraven, Prentice Hall, Inc., Englewood Cliffs, NJ 07632.)

First Degree Heart Block

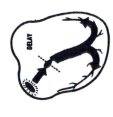

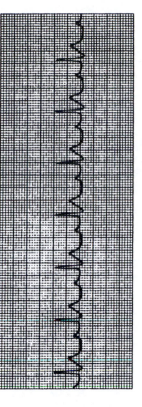

The AV NODE holds each sinus impulse longer than normal before conducting it through the ventricles. Each impulse is eventually conducted. Once into the ventricles, conduction proceeds normally.

REGULARITY: This will depend on the regularity of the underlying rhythm.

RATE: The rate will depend on the rate of the underlying rhythm.

P WAVES: The P waves will be upright and uniform. Each P wave will be followed by a QRS complex.

PRI: The PRI will be constant across the entire strip, but it will always be greater than .20 seconds.

QRS: The QRS complex measurement will be less than .12 seconds.

(Reprinted with permission from *Basic Arrhythmias, 3/E* by Gail Walraven, Prentice Hall, Inc., Englewood Cliffs, NJ 07632.)

Accelerated Junctional Rhythm

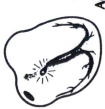

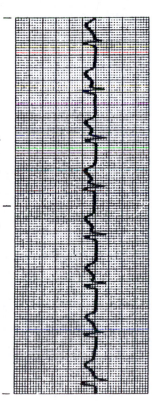

An irritable focus in the AV JUNCTION speeds up to override the SA node for control of the heart. The atria are depolarized via retrograde conduction. Conduction through the ventricles is normal.

REGULARITY: The R–R intervals are constant. The rhythm is regular.

RATE: Atrial and ventricular rates are equal. The rate will be faster than the AV Junction's inherent rate, but not yet into a true tachycardia range. Usually in the 60–100 beats per minute range.

P WAVES: The P wave can come before or after the QRS complex, or it can be lost entirely within the QRS complex. If visible, the P wave will be inverted.

PRI: If the P wave precedes the QRS complex, the PRI will be less than .12 seconds. If the P wave falls within the QRS complex or following it, there will be no PRI.

QRS: The QRS complex will be less than .12 seconds.

(Reprinted with permission from *Basic Arrhythmias, 3/E* by Gail Walraven, Prentice Hall, Inc., Englewood Cliffs, NJ 07632.)

Wenckebach

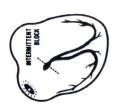

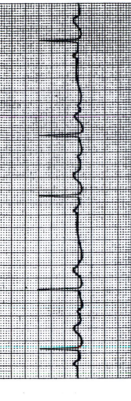

As the sinus node initiates impulses, each one is delayed in the AV NODE a little longer than the preceding one, until one is eventually blocked completely. Those impulses that are conducted travel normally through the ventricles.

REGULARITY: The R–R interval is irregular in a pattern of grouped beating. The R–R interval gets progressively shorter as the PRI gets progressively longer.

RATE: Since some beats are not conducted, the ventricular rate is usually slightly slower than normal. The atrial rate is normal.

P WAVES: The P waves are upright and uniform. Some P waves are not followed by QRS complexes.

PRI: The PR intervals get progressively longer, until one P wave is not followed by a QRS complex. After the blocked beat, the cycle starts again.

QRS: The QRS complex measurement will be less than .12 seconds.

(Reprinted with permission from *Basic Arrhythmias, 3/E* by Gail Walraven, Prentice Hall, Inc., Englewood Cliffs, NJ 07632.)

Classical Second Degree Heart Block

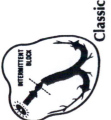

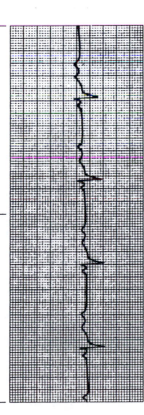

The AV NODE selectively conducts some beats while blocking others. Those that are not blocked are conducted through to the ventricles, although they may encounter a slight delay in the node. Once in the ventricles, conduction proceeds normally.

REGULARITY: If the conduction ratio is consistent, the R–R interval will be constant, and the rhythm will be regular. If the conduction ratio varies, the R–R will be irregular.

RATE: The atrial rate is usually normal. Since many of the atrial impulses are blocked, the ventricular rate will usually be in the bradycardia range, often one half, one third, or one fourth of the atrial rate.

P WAVES: P waves are upright and uniform. There are always more P waves than QRS complexes.

PRI: The PRI on conducted beats will be constant across the strip, although it might be longer than a normal PRI measurement.

QRS: The QRS complex measurement will be less than .12 seconds.

(Reprinted with permission from *Basic Arrhythmias, 3/E* by Gail Walraven, Prentice Hall, Inc., Englewood Cliffs, NJ 07632.)

Premature Atrial Contraction

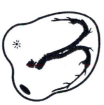

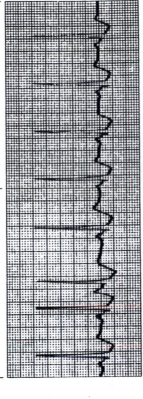

The pacemaker is an irritable focus within the ATRIUM which fires prematurely and produces a single ectopic beat. Conduction through to the ventricles is normal.

REGULARITY: Since this is a single premature ectopic beat, it will interrupt the regularity of the underlying rhythm.

RATE: The overall heart rate will depend on the rate of the underlying rhythm.

P WAVE: The P wave of the premature beat will have a different morphology than the P waves of the rest of the strip. The ectopic beat will have a P wave, but it can be flattened, notched, or otherwise unusual. It may be hidden within the T wave of the preceding complex.

PRI: The PRI should measure between .12 and .20 seconds, but can be prolonged; the PRI of the ectopic will probably be different from the PRI measurements of the other complexes.

QRS: The QRS complex measurement will be less than .12 seconds.

(Reprinted with permission from *Basic Arrhythmias, 3/E* by Gail Walraven, Prentice Hall, Inc., Englewood Cliffs, NJ 07632.)

Complete Heart Block

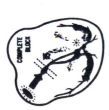

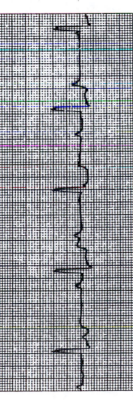

The block at the AV NODE is complete. The sinus beats cannot penetrate the node, and thus, are not conducted through to the ventricles. An escape mechanism from either the junction or the ventricles will take over to pace the ventricles. The atria and the ventricles function in a totally dissociated fashion.

REGULARITY: Both the atrial and the ventricular foci are firing regularly, thus the P–P intervals and the R–R intervals are regular.

RATE: The atrial rate will usually be in a normal range. The ventricular rate will be slower. If a junctional focus is controlling the ventricles, the rate will be 40–60 beats per minute. If the focus is ventricular, the rate will be 20–40 beats per minute.

P WAVES: The P waves are upright and uniform. There are more P waves than QRS complexes.

PRI: Since the block at the AV node is complete, none of the atrial impulses is conducted through to the ventricles. There is no PRI. The P waves have no relationship to the QRS complexes. You may occasionally see a P wave superimposed on the QRS complex.

QRS: If the ventricles are being controlled by a junctional focus, the QRS complex will measure less than .12 seconds. If the focus is ventricular, the QRS will measure .12 seconds or greater.

(Reprinted with permission from *Basic Arrhythmias, 3/E* by Gail Walraven, Prentice Hall, Inc., Englewood Cliffs, NJ 07632.)

Ventricular Tachycardia

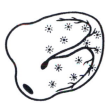

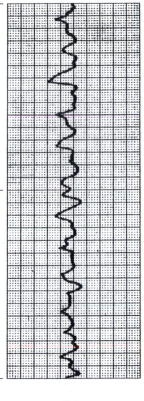

An irritable focus in the VENTRICLES fires regularly at a rate of 150–250 beats per minute to override higher sites for control of the heart.

REGULARITY: This rhythm is usually regular, although it can be slightly-irregular.
RATE: Atrial rate cannot be determined. The ventricular rate range is 150–250 beats per minute. If the rate is below 150 beats per minute it is considered a slow VT. If the rate exceeds 250 beats per minute it's called Ventricular Flutter.
P WAVES: None of the QRS complexes will be preceded by P waves. You may see dissociated P waves intermittently across the strip.
PRI: Since the rhythm originates in the ventricles, there will be no PRI.
QRS: The QRS complexes will be wide and bizarre, measuring at least .12 seconds. It is often difficult to differentiate between the QRS and the T wave.

Ventricular Fibrillation

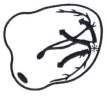

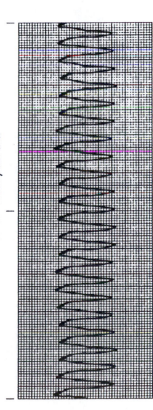

Multiple foci in the ventricles become irritable and generate uncoordinated, chaotic impulses that cause the heart to fibrillate rather than contract.

REGULARITY: There are no waves or complexes that can be analyzed to determine regularity. The baseline is totally chaotic.
RATE: The rate cannot be determined since there are no discernible waves or complexes to measure.
P WAVES: There are no discernible P waves.
PRI: There is no PRI.
QRS: There are no discernible QRS complexes.

Asystole

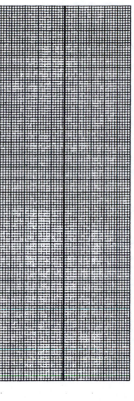

The heart has lost its electrical activity. There is no electrical pacemaker to initiate electrical flow.

REGULARITY: There is no electrical activity; only a straight line.
RATE: There is no electrical activity; only a straight line.
P WAVES: There is no electrical activity; only a straight line.
PRI: There is no electrical activity; only a straight line.
QRS: There is no electrical activity; only a straight line.

(Reprinted with permission from *Basic Arrhythmias, 3/E* by Gail Walraven. Prentice Hall, Inc., Englewood Cliffs, NJ 07632.)

Idioventricular Rhythm

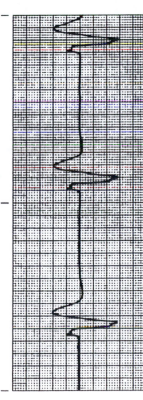

In the absence of a higher pacemaker, the VENTRICLES initiate a regular impulse at their inherent rate of 20–40 beats per minute.

REGULARITY: This rhythm is usually regular, although it can slow as the heart dies.
RATE: The ventricular rate is usually 20–40 beats per minute, but it can drop below 20 beats per minute.
P WAVES: There are no P waves in this arrhythmia.
PRI: There is no PRI.
QRS: The QRS complex is wide and bizarre, measuring at least .12 seconds.

(Reprinted with permission from *Basic Arrhythmias, 3/E* by Gail Walraven, Prentice Hall, Inc., Englewood Cliffs, NJ 07632.)